The Ashley Madison Diaries

The Ashley Madison Diaries

"Sharon Sharalike"

Published by:

AshMad Press

A division of the Ashley Madison Agency®

2300 Yonge Street Suite 2103, P.O. Box 2313
Toronto, Canada M4P 1E4

BURMANBOOKS
.com

BurmanBooks Inc.
4 Lamay Cres. Scarborough,
Ontario Canada • M1X 1J1

This novel is a work of fiction based on the true life experiences of the author. Although it contains incidental references to actual people and places, these references are used to recreate situations upon which the novel is based. All other names, characters, places and incidents have been changed to protect the identities of the parties involved.

graphic design by: ie: Pictures

ISBN: 0-9739097-5-7

Published in Canada
Not for resale

This book is dedicated to my light.
He restored my belief in happily ever after.

Prologue

I went out on my first blind date the summer after my sophomore year at college. I wasn't set up in the usual way by a friend or well-meaning cousin. My favorite cousin, Kate, has made me skeptical of men who are recommended sight unseen, for a date. Kate is a chronic and perpetual dater with a reputation of offering up her latest cast-off to unsuspecting friends and relatives. She once arranged a blind date for her roommate Moira. Moira later confessed to me that the guy Kate had described as "an intensely absorbed conversationalist" turned out to be so boring that five minutes with him gave you a whole new perspective on suicide. Or barring that, mercy killing.

Rather than accept any of my cousin's well-intentioned candidates, who didn't score high enough to rate a second date with her, I found my blind date on my own. I was desperate for that first "Certs encounter". Everyone on campus seemed to be exploring the joys of body contortions with the opposite sex, while I was still trying to find a guy with whom I could attempt to get to first base.

Don't get me wrong, there were lots of cute guys on campus, but the only way I could have gotten their attention was if I'd strapped a neon sign to my chest that said "Free Beer". I'm not ugly, but only by a matter of degrees. I wear glasses so thick that on a sunny day I could start a grass fire by staring at the ground. I'm thin with a flat chest. Sometimes when I catch sight of my reflection in a store window, I look more like Olive Oyl than either of my parents. But unlike the fashion challenged waif, I didn't have a Popeye. Where the hell was he? If Olive Oyl could land a guy with rippling biceps, what was my problem? Even Mini Mouse had Mickey and she was no babe. Have you ever taken a good look at the size of her feet?

I spent my first two years at university waiting for a guy to ask me on a date. At nineteen, my knowledge of the dating scene was limited to what I overheard in the dorm lounge or hallways. When all the girls in my residence got together to bash men, I sat quietly. And when they yapped about the virtues of Matthew, Mark, Luke or John, I listened with the rapt attention of a five-year-old during a favorite bedtime story. Men were a work of fiction to me. They were like Klingons; creatures with a language of their own, which only the insane cared to analyze, a unique, erotically stimulating physique and a set of behavioral patterns so bizarre even Data couldn't figure them out.

By the time I turned twenty, I'd moved past desperate, beyond despair, and had resigned myself to the fact I would never meet a man in a normal way, say at the library, Radio Shack, or Starbucks. I'd traded in my glasses for contacts, and reinvented myself by strictly adhering to the fashion rules dictated by *Vogue*, and *Cosmopolitan*.

No, Mr. Right wouldn't show up at my door with an armful of lilies, a fist full of dollars, and the keys to his Audi 8 swinging seductively from his long, tapered, well-manicured fingers. He didn't exist and even if he did, he probably didn't have a clue how to find my apartment, and, like most men, he was incapable of asking for directions.

The only thing even remotely resembling a man in my life was my roommate Gavin. I had planned to live by myself in a two-bedroom apartment, using the second bedroom for guests or when my parents visited. I found a funky little four-story walk-up. The super of my building had to help me get my stuff up to my third floor unit since there was no elevator. At the time I thought those stairs would be my home gym. Little did I know they'd turn out to be my pain in the ass.

After my first month, I was so cash-strapped I had to get a roommate. That's how Gavin entered my life. We were both in the student union building looking at roommate ads on the bulletin board. He noticed me, introduced himself, and after hearing that I already had a place and was looking for someone to take up the slack rent-wise, volunteered to be that someone. My spider sense warned me about having a guy move into my humble digs. However, I was intrigued by the notion people would think I was shacked up. Gavin seemed harmless. He was my height, if not a smidge shorter. He was also overweight. Not much, just enough to give him a roundish face and one of those potbellies which, while certainly not a turn-on, was kind of cute in a cuddly way.

I guess Gavin noticed I was on the fence about the idea.

In an effort to convince me, he said, "I won't bother you, really. I'm very quiet and practically gay."

"Practically gay? What does that mean?" I asked.

"Well, women don't find me attractive at all, so I never have sex with them. I've never had sex with a guy but, hey, in this day and age, you never know, right? After all, it is the eighties." He was right. It was the eighties. I liked his off-beat humor.

"Why are you so eager to move in with a total stranger?" I asked him. "I could turn out to be a real bitch."

"I've got a good sense about these things. Sort of a spider sense." Spider sense? Me too.

"Besides," he went on, "you're here, I'm here. We're both looking for a roommate and I hate phoning people about big decision stuff like living together. You talk for a bit, agree to meet and then when you do, you have to start discussing arrangements all over again. At least with us, we've already met."

I had to admit, he made sense. Now that he mentioned it, canvassing total strangers on the phone only, then having to meet them was an arduous task. Hmm, maybe that's what I was afraid of when it came to meeting a blind date too. I decided right then and there to be more spontaneous.

"Sure, Gavin. What the hell, you don't look like an ax murderer, and even if you are, I think I could take you. Let's do it."

For the most part, I was pretty happy with him. Aside from the fact that he was a bit of a snoop, and, I suspect, one of those crafty moochers who steals food without leaving incriminating evidence, I didn't regret letting him move in… too much.

Through the power of positive thinking and quick-footedness I managed to avoid most of life's mishaps, blunders, and unappreciated practical jokes. I had reduced my troubles to two main categories: dateless Saturday nights, and declined credit card transactions. So, I took matters into my own capable hands and did what most women in my position would do: I sat down and wrote a Personal ad.

I didn't write my ad alone. I composed it with the help of my two best friends, gin and '7'. If there's a better friend than alcohol, I don't know who it is. My trusty pals never let me down. They help me celebrate the good times, console me during the bad, and when life's circumstances begin to beat me mercilessly into the ground, they offer solace. Did I say solace? I meant to say unconsciousness.

My girlfriend Dakota called me just as I finished writing the first line of my ad. It was unbelievably brilliant. And I'm not just saying that because I wrote it.

"Wanna hear it?" I asked her.

"Sure." she said.

"Winnie the Pooh, where are you?" I waited in breathless anticipation. The big smile melted off my face when anticipation was met with apathy. I waited a little longer for Dakota's response. Still nothing.

"Hello? Dakota? Are you still there?"

"I'm here, but where the hell are you?"

"What do you mean?"

"What kind of ad is that?"

"That's not the whole thing. There's more." I tried to keep the disappointment from my voice.

"Okay, what's the rest?"

"I haven't written it yet." I didn't want to sound defensive, but I probably did.

"All right, give me the basic idea." Dakota kept her voice soft and encouraging.

"Well, I'm hoping to attract some guy who, like, wants to be my teddy bear."

"Hence the allusion to Pooh?"

"Right," I said, snapping my fingers. "You got it."

"I still don't like it." I could almost see Dakota scrunching up her pert nose in distaste.

"What's wrong with it?" How could she not like a headline?

"I think you should have something about who you are and what you're looking for."

"That comes later," I said, wrapping the curly cord of the phone around my arms. It left weird indentations on my skin.

"No," Dakota practically shouted into the phone, "you need that in your headline."

"The headline has to be catchy and interesting."

"That's right." Dakota said this in a tone that made me feel my headline was neither of the above.

"You think my headline is boring?" I was mortified.

"It's not so much boring as sleepy. Know what I mean?"

I didn't know what she meant. I also saw little distinction between "boring" and "sleepy". I thought it was a great headline, but I knew Dakota well enough to know when to pick my fights. Even though I disagreed with her, I gave in anyway.

"Listen, here's what we should do…" she started.

"We? Dakota, when did this become a joint project?"

"The minute you told me about it. Do you want my help or not?"

That was a trick question. I did want her input, but I didn't want her criticism, put-downs, and better-than-thou attitude. Dakota didn't have a boyfriend either, but it was by choice. She was an expert flirt with teeth so luminously perfect, they not only stopped traffic, they could direct it as well. Dakota looked like a cross between Christie Brinkley and Uma Thurman. What more could a guy ask for?

I think Dakota and I had the same basic knowledge of men and machines. In a nutshell, we knew how to turn them on and how to shut them down. The only difference was that Dakota's knowledge about men came from hands-on experience… literally. She had on-the-job training with her McManager. At the end of her shifts, Dakota's uniform was disheveled and untucked. At least I never saw any secret sauce on her shirt. After about three weeks on the job, Dakota received a fifty-cent raise, five times what most employees got. Dakota claimed it was due to her customer service record. I was left wondering what service she was offering and who her customers were.

In spite of this, Dakota was my best friend. Not only did she slip me free fries when I only had enough money for a cheeseburger, she also offered me a shoulder to cry on, when I needed one.

I didn't respond to Dakota's offer of assistance immediately. I wanted someone who could help me word the ad, but I also needed a clear-headed, objective thinker with a creative flair.

Dakota misinterpreted my silence as reluctance. "Stop the presses, I'm coming over."

"You don't have to do that," I said quickly.

"Sure I do. I want to help you." Dakota hung up before I could talk her out of coming over. I got ready for her arrival by pouring myself another drink. I hid my gin bottle behind a red milk crate in my clothes closet. I would've been glad to share my liquor with her, but there were only two-fingers left in the bottle. As it was, I already suspected Gavin was sneaking sips and watering down the rest so I wouldn't know. I had a sixth sense about this sort of thing.

No, there certainly wasn't enough gin to share if I was going to spend Saturday night in an alcohol-induced fog. I put some 7-Up cans in the fridge and salsa and chips on a low wooden table in my living room.

The Brazilian made table made the place look stylish and sophisticated, even though the walls were bare and the living room only had a couch and two bookshelves. I kept my computer in my bedroom, far away from Gavin.

Since the table was the only one in my flat, it had to do triple duty as a coffee table, dining table, and ironing board. The salsa and chips made it a dining table. When Dakota arrived, she dropped her bag on the floor by the front door and brought her clipboard to the table. She stuffed her mouth with the biggest chip in the bowl, and gave me a thumbs-up salute.

"Got anything to drink?" Dakota winked at me.

"Yup." I said, ignoring the wink. I returned with two cans of 7-Up. Dakota was sitting cross-legged at the table. Her clipboard was open and her was mouth full.

"Here you go," I said brightly.

"That's not what I meant," Dakota said frowning at me. I offered the can and she took it.

"Listen, we need to keep clear headed." I warned.

"We also need to be relaxed." Dakota gave me a look. Then added, "Got any Malibu?" I shook my head."Bailey's?"

"No."

"What about Gavin?"

"Listen, I would've been finished with this already if you hadn't invited yourself over." Dakota reflected on this, with her finger in the side of her mouth attempting to dislodge corn chips from her teeth.

Finally she said, "Okay, let's get on with it then." Dakota reached for her clipboard. I handed her a tissue for her fingers. I didn't have any paper towels.

"I have an idea. How's this sound: 'Honey Bear seeks Mr. Sugar Crisp.'"

"I love it!" I said.

"Really?"

"Yes, really."

"Okay. After that we could write: 'Sweet college girl wants special guy for fun and frolic.'"

"No, I don't want frolic in there, because some weird guy is going to think I want to do it with him."

"But you do."

"No, I don't Dakota."

"Sharon, you can't remain a vegan forever!" Dakota refused to say "virgin" since she wasn't one.

"I'm not trying to, I just want to meet a nice guy for dates and whatever."

"The 'whatever' is what I'm trying to work out for you." I hate it when Dakota makes me feel like I'm her charity case, and she has to rescue me from my life.

"How about this," I said, "'College co-ed wants an older guy for...'"

"Fun!" Dakota broke in.

"Okay," I agreed.

"Why do you want an old man?" Dakota dipped another chip and stuck the entire thing in her mouth.

"I don't want an old man. I want someone in fourth-year or a grad student. I'm trying to avoid some pimply freshman."

"Oh..." Dakota's mouth was too full to say anything else. She held up her index finger, which meant wait a minute. When she could speak again she said, "I don't like the word 'old'. You might get Jed Clampett. Use 'mature' instead."

"Okay," I said, grabbing Dakota's clipboard and recording what we had composed through bitter negotiations. I was bitter because the ad was sounding less and less like what I wanted and more and more like what Dakota thought I needed.

We finished the first draft in less than an hour. The chip bowl was empty and the salsa container had been refilled twice. There were crumbs all over the hard wood floor. Dakota always left a mess.

"Okay, I guess my work here is done." Dakota stretched her arms over her head and yawned.

"You could stay and help me clean up." I tried not to sound annoyed.

"Eee, no thanks." Dakota smiled at me like the brilliance of her white teeth would blind me to her laziness.

"Like I said," she continued, "my work here is done." She left without a backward glance. At least I still had my gin and '7'.

I walked around with the ad in my knapsack for a week. Every time Dakota asked me if I'd placed it in the local newspaper, I had to say no. During lunch one afternoon Dakota reached for my bag under the pretense that she needed a pen. She spent the better part of three minutes routing around my books, notepapers, and feminine necessities. I held my breath the entire time.

Finally, she said, "What the hell is this?" She held the scrunched up ad. I looked at her bright green eyes and flushed cheeks. She was livid.

"The thing we worked on," I said, lamely. I didn't want anyone to hear what I knew was about to be a major argument.

"Fuck, Sharon. We went through all that trouble to write this and you still haven't done anything with it?"

"I've been busy. I have to go to classes, you know. I don't have a bunch of adoring admirers taking notes for me."

"Well, you could if you got off your ass and did something for a change."

"I should do something?" I pointed at my chest incredulous. "Aren't you the one who sleeps in till ten, seven days a week?"

"So? I have afternoon classes. If you took your nose out of those friggin' psych books you'd know that."

"You only have afternoon classes so you can party every night."

"Party every night?"

"Yes, that's you, Miss Party Queen." I made my voice high, squeaky and girly in a really bad imitation of Dakota's. "Do you wanna go to a party? There's a Halloween party, wanna go? There's a home coming party, wanna go? There's an 'I'm-so-pretty party,' wanna go?" I changed back to my normal voice, and said emphatically, "I'm tired of going to those stupid parties. I've had it up to here with holding your drink and looking after your coat. Okay?"

"Listen b…" I'm pretty sure Dakota was going to say "bitch", but she caught herself at the last second, rearranged her sentence, and her face. "Buddy. I do all that for you. You think I'm having a good time going out every fucking Thursday, Friday, and Saturday night?"

"Yes," I said smugly. I crossed my hands across my chest because I could feel victory, but I couldn't high five myself.

"I've worked so hard to help you get out of your self-imposed exile. And you know what? After today, I'm finished. If you wanna spend the rest of your life a bitter spinster because you are 5' 7" instead of 5' 9", unhappy because your tits aren't huge, lonely because you don't have the guts to get out there and try something new, then be my guest. This is your life; I can't live it for you. You're in control of your own destiny."

"I know that."

"I guess that's why this is still in here." Dakota held up the scrunched paper. She put it back in my knapsack. I took my bag from her and she didn't resist. We sat for a moment in total silence. I could tell that people around us were riveted, waiting for round two to begin. I felt like I'd had the wind knocked out of my sails. I was hurt and angry and disappointed in myself for disappointing Dakota. I knew she wanted me to get out there and meet people, primarily guys. I knew she meant well, but it felt utterly pointless.

Dakota got up from the table and gathered her stuff. I could tell she thought I was a loser. "At this rate," she said, "you're going to be a vegan for the rest of your life!" She walked out of the cafeteria with at least twenty-six pairs of eyes on her.

On my way from the cafeteria, a guy who'd heard what Dakota had said, stopped me and offered half his ham sandwich. I was going to say no, but he had such an earnest face I changed my mind and

I took it. I even took a bite in front of him.

"This is good," I said.

"If you like that, wait till you try turkey."

"That's what I'm afraid I'll get," I shot back. I left too disheartened to explain I was talking about men.

It took me another three days to find the time to place the ad. (Read "work up the courage.") All I had to do was fill out the form and mail it to the *Tribune*. After that, someone would call me with a mailbox number and code. Anyone responding to my ad would leave a message in my mail account, then all I had to do was use my special code to retrieve messages. Simple right? Well no, not for me. I had Gavin for a roommate.

I had to keep all things private and personal from him. If he picked up the message from the newspaper about my mailbox number and special secret code, he'd know what I was up to. Plus he could access my messages. I couldn't sit by the phone for the next two days waiting for the paper to call. The only thing I could do was place the ad in person and retrieve my code there and then.

I got to the *Tribune* building without a hitch, if you ignore that I missed my bus and had to wait three-quarters-of-an-hour for the next one. The building lobby was about two stories high, with beige marble floors and matching walls. I had no idea where to go, so I headed straight toward the impressive looking information desk. Behind it sat a security guard dressed in black. He looked more like a secret service agent than a security guard. I approached his desk and leaned on it like it was the counter in a candy store.

"Can I help you?" The guard wore a vacant expression, but his voice was velvety like chocolate.

"Yes, I want the, um, ad department." I was placing an ad right? So that had to be the department I needed.

"Third floor," he said, without looking at me. He was focused on something just over my head.

"Thanks," I said.

"The elevator banks are to your left." I was headed to the right and had to do an about-face without losing my balance. I smiled as I passed the guard. He just stared at me like I was from Venus.

When I got to the third floor there was a smaller desk, but it was just as intimidating as the first. Behind this one was a woman, small with dark hair and round, John Lennon glasses.

"Yes," a frosty cold voice barked.

"I want to place a Personal ad."

"A whot?" British accent. Not a good sign. She sounded like James Bond's secretary. Abort mission, turn around, retreat.

My feet remained planted and I heard myself say,"An ad for the Personal section of the paper."

"I beg your pardon? I'm afraid I don't understand."

"I just want to place this ad in your paper in the Personals."

"I don't believe we have anything of the sort."

"You do," I shot back. This Moneypenny bitch made me feel both shaken and stirred.

"One moment." She picked up the phone and used bony fingers to punch in a four-digit number that began with two and ended with nine although it looked like six from where I was standing. Then she said, "There's someone here about a Personal ad." She said "Personal ad" the way AA members say virgin cocktail. This was followed by a few "oohs," and a "very well then," and an "I shall." Then she hung up the phone and placed her two hands together to form a bridge.

"You need Community Services. It's in the basement." She said basement in a funny way, but I thanked her just the same. I retreated to the elevators. Thankfully, one of the elevators opened the minute I pressed the button. I hopped on quickly, and pressed the close-door key like my life depended on it.

When I got to the basement, another desk awaited me. It was small and shabby, with one broken leg. It reminded me of the kind grade-school teachers have. There was no one behind it, so I rang the bell.

A voice called out, "I'm coming, wait please." The guy appeared with lots of dusty papers in his hands. He dropped them on the desk.

"What can I do you for?"

"I want to place an ad."

"Garage sale?"

"No, something for the Personals."

"Okay, how many lines have you got?"

"Six," I said, glad to be speaking to someone who could actually help me.

"All right, that will be nine dollars."

"Nine dollars? I thought this was free!"

"The first three lines are free; after that it's $2.95 per line."

"Well, can I just do three lines then?"

"Sure can." He handed me a ballpoint pen. I had to pare down the ad on the spot. I crossed out several words, rearranged some, and drew a squiggly line through the rest. I handed over my crumpled paper.

"Okay, three dollars."

"What do you mean, three dollars? I only have three lines."

"Your headline counts as a line." I took the sheet from him swearing under my breath. I crossed out more words and handed it back.

"Looks good," he said slapping the limp paper with his left hand.

"Do you think I could have the code to retrieve my mail now?"

"You're anticipating a lot of mail, eh?" He gave me a wink and a conspiratorial nod, which I ignored.

"It's easier if I just get it now."

"Okay then, coming right up. Give me a moment." The moment he requested turned into twenty-three long minutes. But when he finally returned, he gave me my mailbox number, as it would appear in the newspaper, and my secret code for retrieving my mail.

"Good luck" he said, as I turned to leave.

"Thanks," I said, smiling for the first time since my fight with Dakota.

The Personals appeared in the Tuesday edition. I placed my ad on a Wednesday morning, so I had to wait almost an entire week to see it. I got up early that Tuesday and left home before nine. I bought a paper from a vending box and took two since there was no one around. I took both papers home. Gavin was in the kitchen. I raced to my room with just a quick, "Good morning." I didn't wait for his response, which was likely to be a curse anyway. Gavin was not a morning person. Once I was safely in my bedroom, I flipped to the Personals, throwing the rest of the paper aside. The ads were listed alphabetically under the heading Women seeking Men. As soon as I spotted mine, I called Dakota.

"Hello?" Dakota's voice was thick with sleep.

"My ad's in the paper." I said in a hushed tone. I kept my voice just above a whisper so Gavin wouldn't hear. An ear-piercing scream ensued.

"Sharon, I'm so happy for you. I can't believe you did it."

"I can't believe it either. Do you think there are any messages yet?"

"There could be. I'm coming over. Don't check your mailbox until I get there."

"Okay," I agreed. I was already reaching for my secret code. It was in my wallet.

"I think this is going to change your life," Dakota said. She was so positive about everything. Maybe that's why good things always seemed to find her. But this time, I kept my thoughts positive too, and look what happened to me. I met Dogbiscuit and boy, did he ever change my life.

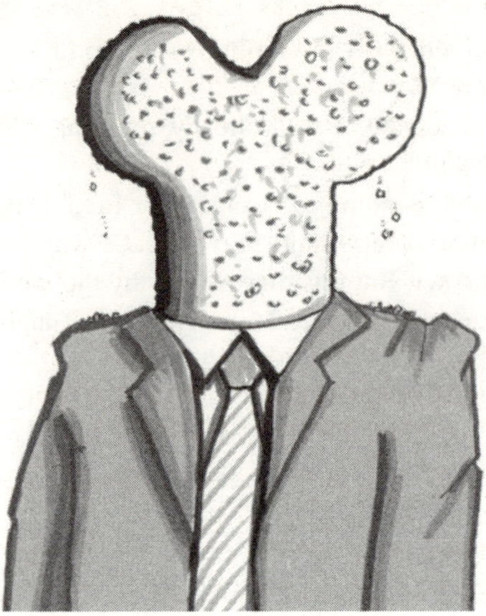

Chapter One:
Dogbiscuit

When I woke up, I could hear the shower going. I tried to open my eyes, but failed because the sheer white curtains were no match for the brilliance of the morning sun. Without opening my eyes, I rummaged around my bedside table to find an Air Canada eye mask I'd received in this really lovely toiletry purse when I flew first class to Bermuda. My hand slipped across lip balm, my diary, cuticle cream, a nail file, a leather bookmark, cuticle scissors, a note pad and a pen for recording my dreams. A T-tag slipped up under my nail.

"Shit." I squeezed my eyes tighter shut. I finally found the eye mask jammed against the back of the drawer. I pulled on the string and it came out along with a nail clipper I thought I'd lost. I put the mask on and let the nail clipper fall back into the drawer.

I tried to settle back to sleep, but the shower had stopped and the next round of noises from the bathroom set my teeth on edge. Retching sounds were followed by a few coughs, a sputter, and a gag.

Then the faucet was going, full throttle. An electric razor came on next. Then some loud tapping. This was followed by another round of retching, and a few boisterous gargles. A bit of projectile spitting ended the set. I was lulled to sleep.

"Why do you have that damn thing on your face?" It was Dogbiscuit. He didn't normally talk to me, but when he did, I was usually on the phone or unconscious.

"Are you awake?"

"I am now," I said grumpily.

"Why do you have that mask on? You look like a super hero who took a wrong turn and ended up here." I lifted a corner of the patch and glared at him. He was starring back at me with his big brown eyes. Not the teddy bear kind, no, his eyes were like tiger-eyes, cool and assessing with yellow centers. Once I thought they were sexy because they could be deep pools of brown or yellow when his mood changed. Now he looked to me like a predator. He was a wolf in Hugo Boss clothing.

"Were you drinking last night? You look bloody awful. Look at your eyes; they're puffy and red like those God awful cherries in your mother's yard."

"They're red from lack of sleep, which is what this mask is for." I released the corner and adjusted the mask firmly over my face. I didn't want to look at him standing over me with his black coffee in one hand and his morning newspaper in the other. And I definitely didn't want to see any more of his $1500 navy suit, with his perfectly coordinated blue camouflage tie. His shiny black hair reflected the sun's rays made my head throb. Honestly, does the captain of industry really need so much pomade? Dogbiscuit is single handedly responsible for half of Brill Cream's annual revenues.

"So, the mask is really for me?" Without looking, I could tell he was using his newspaper hand to point to himself."Well thanks, I guess it saves me from having to look at those sore eyes." As if he ever looked at me.

"Can you please shut up and let me get some sleep?" The only reason he was talking to me was because he was jealous. I could sleep till eight and he had to be out of the house by seven-thirty.

I could tell he was still starring at me. I kept my mask on, while I sat up and rearranged the sheets. I try not to touch his side of the bed, and he stays away from mine. "Okay, Zorro," I heard him say. "Just don't carve your initials into the bed." This was followed by stomping feet. A few minutes later the front door creaked open, then slammed shut. I took a deep breath and then exhaled.

Living with Dogbiscuit wasn't horrible, although it was a challenge. I'd lived with worse. Gavin was no treat of the week, but he did pay two-thirds of the rent. Dogbiscuit pays the mortgage. If I have learned anything from living with those two, it has to be that life is about compromise, sacrifice and survival. The only thing is, I'm not sure I can survive life with Dogbiscuit.

I married Dogbiscuit when I gave up on finding Prince Charming. I was also six months pregnant and didn't feel I could pull off the Murphy Brown routine. So we tied the knot, even though Kate said it was bad luck to marry the first guy you sleep with, and Dakota said, "Place another ad and this time leave out the word mature."

Oh that fateful ad! I did get a lot of responses, just like Dakota had predicted. The only problem was that most of the men were from the Rat Pack Era. The kind of guys who'd call Paul Newman a kid. When did mature become synonymous with ancient? One guy who called actually had those vocal tremors old people get. His voice was all quivery, and he could barely hear me. After everything I said he'd ask, "What was that?" or "Come again?" Well, come was the one thing I knew I wouldn't do with grandpa.

Most of the men who answered my ad said they were in their forties which means they were pushing sixty hard. I used the word "mature" in the ad because I thought it would attract fourth-year students. I was hoping for a guy working on his business degree. Ideally, he'd have one foot on the corporate ladder and the other tangled in my bed sheets. Instead, I ended up with men so old they had one foot in the grave and the other soaking in Ben Gay.

I don't know what those men were thinking when they left messages in the box of a twenty-year-old. "Sex is what they were thinking. Pure unadulterated sex." That's what Dakota had said. But she has a one-track mind, so I'm not sure she really got what those men were all about. Nor did I. I never understood what they thought we'd do together. I mean, can you imagine a geriatric trying to master inline skates with his walker?

Patrick was the only man I agreed to meet. He was charming,

sweet and insisted we get together. I didn't have the heart to say no. Plus Dakota thought I could get a free lunch out of it, but in the end Patrick and I decided to meet for coffee. I couldn't really come up with anything he could do, being so old. We set the date for a Thursday afternoon. I was excited and terrified all at once. I tried to keep myself from becoming too hopeful. After all, I knew he was old and it wasn't likely that we would make a love connection. Despite the dismal prognosis, I dressed for success. I wore a short black skirt, tall boots, and a baby blue V-neck sweater. Patrick showed up in pants that were belted a little under his chest bone, and a striped, short-sleeve, lime-green shirt. Sadly, this was before lime-green had made a come back. I smiled at him and he came over to with his arms outstretched.

"Sharon?"

"Hi Patrick," I said, getting a good look at his face.

He had just enough gray hair to make him look like those principals who think they're in touch with their student body. In reality, they're barely in touch with themselves. Patrick's handshake was firm and so strong, I knew he could beat just about anybody in an arm wrestle.

"How did you spot me so quickly?" Although his question was sincere, if he'd looked around the room he would've found the answer written on the faces of every co-ed in the place. The donut shop was just outside the college grounds, so naturally it was a hangout for everyone trying to avoid the campus scene. It was full of third and fourth year students. In that environment, Patrick looked like the ghost from Christmas Past. I shrugged my shoulders in answer to Patrick's question.

"Just a lucky guess," I said lamely.

"Shall we?" Patrick made a gesture toward the chairs by the window. We sat at a gritty round table. It was wobbly, but Patrick didn't seem to notice. He was staring at me. "You are very, very, pretty," he said.

"Thanks," I said, turning away to look at the donuts stacked along the wall behind the counter. I was flattered by Patrick's compliment. Dakota had insisted on giving me a make-over for my date. I was wearing plum eyeshadow and soft pink lip gloss. Even I had to admit that I looked nice. Dakota wanted me to cut my hair. She thought I'd look like Courtney Cox in the Bruce Springstein video. I wasn't sure she was right, but if she was, I might not have to waste my time eating donuts with sexagenarians. I returned my attention to Patrick. He was opening his mouth to speak. It's weird how old people move so slowly. It was like watching a film in slow motion.

"What can I get for you?" He said this in a really grand way, like if I'd said, "I'll have a BMW and a house in the hills" he'd get it for me without breaking a sweat.

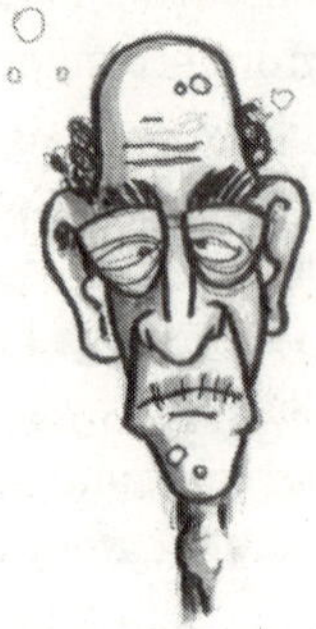

"Can you get me a milk, and a chocolate donut?" I asked, returning my gaze to his face. Maybe I'd try the BMW and the house later.

"Of course," he said, bowing slightly. He went up to the counter and I couldn't help but notice how steady he was on his feet. What made me think he'd need a walker? The only old thing about him was how slowly he seemed to be moving. It was as if he was walking in slow motion. When Patrick returned, he brought tea in a styrofoam cup, the milk I had ordered and a donut with chocolate icing. I'd wanted a chocolate donut, but I just said thank you.

"That's what you wanted, right?" I nodded. "Good, I was afraid I would bring you chocolate milk and a jelly donut." Patrick laughed as if he'd made a really witty remark. Even though he wasn't as old as I'd expected, it was probably a real effort for him to keep things organized in his mind. I'd read in my psychology book that dementia was a characteristic of aging.

"So what do you do for fun?"

"I mostly read, ride my bike, run, that sort of thing," I answered.

"Ah, yes, I remember you telling me you like a lot of sports."

"You like golf, right?" I remembered he'd said that his favorite sports were golf and tennis. I could get into tennis, but golf clothes are really wretched.

"That's right, you remembered." Patrick seemed really pleased by that. I smiled and he smiled back. The only difference was when I smiled you saw white teeth. Not white like Xerox paper, but they looked good. When Patrick smiled, it was like looking at a broken-down fence on a farm in Mississippi. No two teeth were headed in the same direction. Every tooth in his mouth had its own agenda and alignment didn't figure into it. I was so stunned, my smile turned into a "What the hell?" look. Patrick must have read my expression because he looked over his shoulder.

"Is something the matter?"

"No," I said quickly, shaking my milk carton. *Just don't smile again,* I thought. I opened my milk and took a long gulp.

"I should have brought you a straw."

"It's okay," I said, reaching for a napkin to remove my milk mustache.

"I'll get you one." Patrick got up before I could say anything further. Fine, get a straw. He was such a pleaser. When we talked on the phone he told me his wife had divorced him, probably because if she stuck around, he would've smothered her with his I'll-take-care-of-you routine.

By the time Patrick returned with the straw, I'd finished my donut, and half the milk was gone. I used the straw anyway. Then I had to sit and watch Patrick drink his tea. I didn't like the way he pursed his lips over the cup. Your lips don't have to be such a major part of drinking tea. Just bring the cup to your mouth and pour it in. Lips don't have to meet the cup halfway. While Patrick drank his tea, we talked about nothing. Which is to say he told me about playing in a golf tournament, then he complained about the crummy weather, and the lousy public transit.

"Don't you drive?" I asked.

"Yes, but I was thinking of how tough it must be for you to get around."

"Oh," I said. Well that was kind of sweet. He was a nice man.

"I know I'm too old for you but…" his voice trailed off.

What's with the "but?" You're too old for me period. There is no "but."

"Oh, you're not that old," I said, trying to sound as sincere as possible. Patrick took another sip of his tea and I guess he swallowed the wrong way because he made one of those half-cough/half-chokes and spit some tea on his lap.

"Well," I said, ready to end things diplomatically, "it was great to have met you." I reached my hand across the table for the friendship handshake. To my absolute horror, he pulled my arm toward his body, leaned forward and kissed me on the cheek. His lips were warm and wet, as if he was holding tea in his mouth. I was so appalled, I wanted to dry my cheek and slap his face, but I didn't want to offend him. I got up from the table, careful not to knock it over. "Thanks for the milk and donut. 'Bye." I waved at him with my palm out, the way you gesture toward a dog when commanding it to stay. I was hoping he'd get the hint. He didn't.

"Oh Sharon, would you like me to drive you home?"

"It's not that far. I'm going to walk."

"Are you sure? It's really no trouble."

"That's okay. I like to walk." Which was true, I do like to walk, I just didn't normally enjoy walking alone.

"Well can I call you again?"

"Sure," I said, nodding my head while backing away. I wanted to turn and run, but I didn't want to be rude. So I just waved again and walked out calmly. My brain was screaming, *That man put his saliva on my face!* But I just kept walking slowly, willing myself to stay calm. When I couldn't see the donut shop anymore, I pulled a Kleenex from my bag and scrubbed at my cheek until it was numb.

When I got home, Gavin was in the living room watching TV. He looked up at me and held his hand out in a halt salute. "Not a word from you," he said. "I don't care what you've bought or what your score was on your latest test. I'm watching my show. Oh by the way, who socked you in the face?"

"Gavin, can you please not intrude into my personal affairs?" I kept walking past him toward my bedroom.

"Have you had a lover's quarrel? Oops, I forgot you don't have a lover. Well, whoever mucked up your face can be punished. I'll kick the crap out of him for you… But not until my show ends."

I slammed my bedroom door, went into my washroom and examined my cheek. All the rubbing had made it look sore. I washed my face. It would look better soon. I turned the light off in the bathroom, walked over to my neatly made bed and belly-flopped onto the purple sheets. Gavin had the TV volume at full blast, but oddly enough, I couldn't make out what was being said. The speaking pattern of the actors sounded like a soap opera. Gavin loved soaps and game shows. He never watched the news or documentaries. His theory was that the news was filled with propaganda and subliminal mind controlling messages. According to Gavin, the subliminal messages were responsible for all those fires in Tonawanda.

I put one of my pillows over my head to block out the incessant white noise. When that failed, I got up and grabbed my phone off the dresser. I called Dakota, and told her about Patrick. She tried to tell me it couldn't have been all that bad, but she hadn't seen Patrick's teeth!

When I mentioned this, Dakota said, "He was basically a nice person, you just didn't like his teeth. Right?"

"Yes, but I don't think I want to go out on any more blind dates."

"Why not? You're going to let one bad experience turn you off?"

"Yes. You don't understand; everyone responding to my ad is so old."

"Wait another week. I'm sure someone better will turn up."

Indeed the calls kept coming. One after the other. I rejected each respondent. When final exams started, I didn't have time to deal with any of this any more and finally had to pull the plug on the ad. I put men on the back burner again. When I wasn't even thinking about men, I met Dogbiscuit.

I was on my way to the gymnasium, where I was scheduled to take a computer science exam. There were about 600 students. I was so nervous, I left my brand new pen and pencil set on my bed. I used new pens for every exam because they haven't made any mistakes yet. I know it's a silly superstition, but it works for me.

I'd started rooting through my purse when this guy came over and asked, "Need a pen?"

I looked down at him, because he was at least two inches shorter than me and I said, "Do you have one?"

"You can borrow this one." I took it with the promise to return it after the exam. My exam was over before his, so I had to sit in the sun and wait for him. When he finally came out, he greeted me with a big smile. Clean white teeth, nicer than mine. Well, not really nicer, but almost.

"My pen?' he asked.

"Here you go, thanks a lot." I could look up at him since I was sitting down. I used my right hand as a visor. I thought he would take his pen and leave, but he sat down beside me.

"That was my last exam," he said pulling grass up and tossing it in front of his short legs.

"Lucky you," I said.

"How many have you got left?"

"A lot. I'm only in second year."

"Really?"

"Yup." I nodded at him for emphasis.

His left eyebrow went up. "You look older," he said, and I felt flattered.

"I do?"

"Yeah." Now he nodded at me.

"Well, thanks." I smiled. That was the best compliment I'd heard in a long time.

"I thought you were a graduate student. There's something really old about you." That was Dogbiscuit for you, first he gave you a compliment, then he took it away. Despite his lack of charm, there was something likeable about him, although it took me years to finally put my finger on it, and when I did, it dissipated. He asked me to have lunch with him the following week. I agreed. A week after that, he invited me to a movie. It was *To Live and Die in LA*. I thought it was a little violent for a first date flick, but hey, it was dark and I was sitting next to a man. Two out of three ain't bad. After the movie, we went for coffee and dessert. Even though he didn't say very much, I had a great time talking about the film. Can you blame me? I love talking about movies, and he was a good listener.

Three months after we met, we had dinner at the Four Seasons. When he told me he'd reserved a room for us, I thought he was the most sophisticated man in the world. After dinner, I was too liquored-up from the Crystal to give more than a fleeting thought to the fact that I didn't have a toothbrush or a change of underwear. I also hadn't really thought about losing my virginity. But if it had to go, could there be a better place than the Four Seasons hotel? Not likely.

The night we spent at the Four Seasons was the most romantic thing Dogbiscuit ever did. Our relationship was strictly downhill from that moment on. I should have left him, but I got so used to having someone to share movies and the cost of groceries with, that I stayed. And besides, I thought that by staying with Dogbiscuit, I could avoid those lonely feelings that would creep up on me when I saw couples doing the most mundane things, like holding hands at a stop light. When I thought about my own parents and how well they fit together, like white bread and honey, or macaroni and cheese, I had yearnings for a special someone of my own. I wanted the peanut butter that would compliment my jelly, the cream for my coffee. I didn't want to give Dogbiscuit up, even though I knew from the very beginning that he wasn't right for me. I knew I didn't love him. But with him, I had so much more than I had without him. And when he was around I felt like we were one of those couples I used to envy.

But the number one reason I stayed with Dogbiscuit was because having him in my life meant I never had to place another ad in a second-rate newspaper, go out on a blind date with any of the Geritol set, or spend another Saturday night alone. At least that's what I thought at the time. So, I allowed a stupid Bic pen to bring Dogbiscuit into my life. Then I became pregnant, and suddenly, all my reasons for staying with Dogbiscuit took a back seat to a more sincere sense of duty. When I got pregnant, I started to see Dogbiscuit for the person he really was. After I told him I was pregnant, he immediately became distant. I'll give him credit, he said all the right things: "I'll support whatever decision you make," "Don't worry, I'll do right by you" and "I'm here for you." But the way he said it was about as sincere as Bill Clinton's testimony during his impeachment trial. I wondered if Dogbiscuit was advised to say those things to protect any possible future career in politics. Six months later, I was married in a civil ceremony. It was a far cry from the wedding of my dreams. I didn't have eight bridesmaids with matching grooms. And I wasn't ushered to the church in a Rolls Royce limousine. In fact, at the very moment I was counting out my bus fare, my father called me. He wanted to know how I was getting to the city hall. I didn't want to tell him I was taking the bus. Dogbiscuit was too occupied with his own misery to worry about me. My father is nobody's fool. After a few probing questions he guessed the situation and thirty-five minutes before I was due to meet Dogbiscuit, my parents arrived at my apartment and whisked me away to my doom.

When we arrived at city hall, Dogbiscuit's parents were already sitting in the civil ceremonies room. They looked equally miserable. I had the sense that Dogbiscuit's parents blamed me for the pregnancy. It was obvious to everyone that they thought I was using maternity as my pathway to marriage. I wasn't. I never wanted to be married. Of course I had fantasies about falling in love with James Bond, but I never imagined myself as a wife. I was still trying to figure out how to become a good girlfriend.

I didn't gain any comfort from my own parents. They wore their dislike for Dogbiscuit like Halloween masks. My father's scowl was no match for the deep crevices of my mother's frown. I wanted to reassure them that he was kind and decent, but I had no evidence of this. He seemed to me to be singular in his pursuits, inflexible in his habits, and stingy in all matters pertaining to me.

While we waited for the justice of the peace to arrive, my father actually attempted to apologize for not protecting me better. He saw Dogbiscuit as the evil defiler who'd ruined his beloved daughter. I glanced across the room at Dogbiscuit and his parents. They had only expressed a perfunctory greeting when we'd arrived. I tried to smile, but Dogbiscuit's mother fixed me with a look so vicious I knew she wouldn't be joining us for the Chinese Buffet luncheon my own mother had thought would be grand.

The worst part of the ceremony was when Dogbiscuit was asked if he took me to be his lawfully wedded wife. He exhaled such a resigned sigh before uttering a very reluctant, "I do," that I knew he didn't love me and never would. He was acting as though he was Superman and I was kryptonite.

I was so hurt, I was ready to speak up when the justice of the peace asked if there was anyone who objected to the marriage. Then I had a flash of raising an infant by myself in my cramped little apartment with Gavin constantly mooching jars of baby food. I remained quiet.

Dogbiscuit and I never had a honeymoon. After the buffet, which his parents did not attend, I went home with my parents. I'm not sure where Dogbiscuit went. He said he had to make some arrangements. This turned out to be buying a house in Forest Hill. I didn't hear from Dogbiscuit for two days. On the third day, he called to say he and his mother had found us a house.

The house was situated on Prince William Drive. It was a gorgeous two-story Victorian, with a center hall. I loved the house from the moment I saw it. I should have been offended that I was excluded from the purchase, but I wasn't. I was secretly thrilled when Dogbiscuit drove the Budget van onto the circular drive. I didn't dare show excitement lest I be accused of trapping a husband for the trappings of a house.

Before I had a chance to hang anything in my walk-in closet, Dogbiscuit presented me with a post-nuptial agreement. Essentially I was being asked to sign away all spousal rights to the house,

Dogbiscuit's stocks, bonds, and his money master account, the value of which I knew nothing about. I signed this in good faith, without the presence of a lawyer, to prove once and for all, I was not after Dogbiscuit's money. Dogbiscuit told me he was mortgaged up to his eye teeth and he wanted to make sure he didn't lose everything. I signed my name with a flourish. I was certain the contract was his mother's idea. She seemed to think her son was heir to the throne and I was Fergie.

Three-and-a-half months after we'd moved into our home in Forest Hill, I gave birth to a seven pound baby girl. I named her Mackenzie. Two years later, I had another baby. It was a boy I called Connor. I gave my children solid Irish names to impress their paternal grandmother. Unfortunately, she never seemed to notice the effort I'd made to honor her. However, she did seem to delight in her grandchildren in a brittle sort of way.

I enjoyed being a mother, although I kept looking for a manual in bookstores. It was the toughest job I'd ever had. Well no, actually being Dogbiscuit's wife was far more challenging.

At best, my marriage was a lonely institution, at worst it was a turbulent nightmare that made me cry myself to sleep, even though I had things in my life that should have brought me happiness.

I felt like a prisoner who'd been cast away on a deserted island. I was all set to live out my life sentence, longing for the day my kids left for college, so I could leave with them. Then a peculiar thing happened. I was out with Dakota at Sassafrass, our favorite hangout, not including retail stores, when she told me she had a solution to my problem.

"You have a Stepford husband for me?" I asked sipping my green apple martini, grateful that someone recognized my plight and wanted to do something about it.

"Better," Dakota said grinning from ear to ear. She pulled a small bit of newspaper from her black Kate Spade purse and handed it to me. It was from the classified section and at a glance I could tell this was about blind date encounters. I shook my head as an image of Patrick came to mind, namely his peanut teeth.

"Don't even go there. I've been there, and done that."

"No, no, no. You don't get it. This is about using the Internet." The way she said Internet was like the way some people said UFO-Files.

"Listen to me, Dakota, if this has anything to do with meeting men, I'm not interested. I already have Dogbiscuit to deal with, every fucking day. Do you really think I need more bullshit in my life?"

"It's precisely because you are yoked to that asshole that I saved this for you." I took the scrap of newspaper from Dakota. She was drinking a chocolate mocha martini, which she swore up and down tasted like a brownie. Right. She looked at me over the rim until I bent my head and read the clipping I held between my French manicured fingers.

The heading was: The Ashley Madison Agency. It was written in fancy letters that looked elegant or sexy, depending on whether you're reading a tasteful romance novel or a steamy erotic thriller. There was a picture of a woman whispering to a really hot guy. A married woman, a woman like me, with unmet needs, and a desire for something more. After I'd read everything printed in the box, I looked up. Dakota was grinning at me with clasped hands.

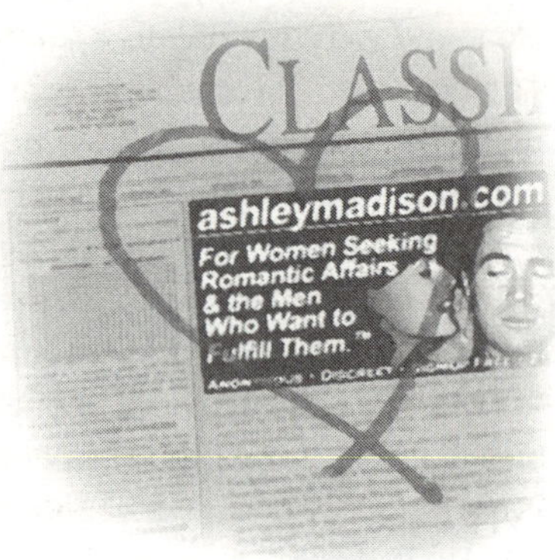

"Well? Do you want to do it?"

"No," I said, handing the paper back to her.

"You're crazy! This is your way out. This is the answer to your prayers."

"How do you figure an affair is going to help me?"

"It'll take your mind off Dogbiscuit." We both giggled.

"Look Dakota, I know you mean well, but uh, no. No thank you."

"Why not? Why can't you just try it?"

"Because I don't want to."

"What are you afraid of?"

"I'm not afraid of anything. I just don't want to do it."

"What if you met someone and he made you feel alive? What if you met someone and he made you laugh out loud?"

"Why, because he dressed badly?"

"No, because he made you feel happy." I didn't have a witty come back for that one, so I stayed quiet.

"What if you met someone and he made you so happy that when you sighed you said his name."

"Why, are there a lot of long vowels in it?"

"Listen you can wise crack the rest of your life away, chained to a man you don't love, and trying to spend quality time with kids who are so busy, you have to book their bedtime story three weeks in advance." Was my life that dismal?

"Or," Dakota continued using her sexiest voice like she was trying to seduce me, "you can take a chance on having a discreet, long-term affair, with a man who, like you, plans to stay married, but wants a little something on the side. Maybe someone to help with the winter blues, or someone to quench your thirst on those hot summer nights."

"You know what I'd really like?"

"What?" Dakota drank her martini then licked her lips like it really did taste like a brownie.

"I would like to meet someone who'd tell me that I'm beautiful."

"You are beautiful, you don't need a man for that. I'm always telling you how great you look." It was true. Dakota had finally convinced me that I did look good. I was wearing my hair short in a style that made my almond-shaped eyes look too big for my face, while my lips took on a pout that was so full I could have been the next Revlon spokesmodel. My two pregnancies had left their mark in the measured tones of 36-25-36. My AA breasts filled out during pregnancy to an astonishing C-cup. So determined was I to hang onto those new breasts, that I'd made a solemn decision to breast feed Connor until he was eight. This resolution ended the moment Connor started chewing on my nipples. The pain was so searing it sent shivers up my spine and all the way to the roots of my hair. I had to relent and introduce solid food. Fortunately, my breasts diminished only slightly. When all my milk was gone, I was still left with two impressive B-cup breasts with nipples that pointed forward instead of down.

I could no longer be mistaken for Olive Oyl. When I stood naked in front of the floor-length mirror in my bedroom, I was amazed to find my head sitting on top of Betty Boop's body.

Don't think I took my new body for granted, because I didn't. I am committed to its wellness. I work out every chance I get even if those chances only come after I've gorged on a bag of Doritos and a tub of Ben & Jerry's *Dolce Vita*.

"I know I don't need a man to tell me I'm beautiful, but that's what I want. I want someone who makes me feel desirable and sexy."

"In other words, you're still looking for Prince Charming."

"Yes," I said, conveying defeat with my slumped shoulders. Behind the walls of my false bravado, I was still looking for Mr. Everything. I'm twenty-eight years old, unhappily married to a man who can't spare five minutes to talk to me, and I still believe in fairy tales. I have to, because the idea that somewhere out there is a man who might actually be my soulmate, my better half, the love of my life, is what keeps me going. It's that tiny glimmer of hope that gets me through those long, lonely nights, when all I'm thinking is, *wouldn't it be nice to have someone's hand to hold.* Or when I think about what it would feel like to fall asleep in the arms of the man I love, and wake up cradled in his embrace.

Sometimes I think that life without love is like taking poison. The kind that dries you up and turns you into one of those pinched, sour-faced women you see behind the wheels of super-sized luxury SUVs. They compensate for the lack of love in their lives with bigger cars, glittery diamonds, Donna Karan clothing, Gucci sunglasses, Prada shoes, and cruises to Alaska. Wait a minute, maybe that life isn't such a bad gig. I wouldn't mind a precious thing or two. But then Dakota had a lot of material wealth and she didn't seem particularly ecstatic.

Don't get me wrong. It's not that Dogbiscuit is so bad. It's just that he's not so good. He's not abusive, in the traditional way soccer players and rock stars beat up their wives. Rather, he's the kind who's guilty of negligence. I've tried to get him to notice me, but nothing has worked. He never noticed when Sabatino cut my hair. Dakota was certain Dogbiscuit would love it. If he did, he kept this information to himself.

After the hair cut, I tried to dress sexier. I was a stay-at-home mom who wore leotards when I wasn't wearing yoga pants. This didn't seem to do anything to spark Dogbiscuit's interest in me, so I modified my wardrobe. I got rid of everything with lycra, a move I later regretted, and bought several short skirts, funky tops, and flared pants. Kate helped me with the jewelry. She made me exchange my pearl earrings for white gold hoops. I bought matching bangles too. They jingled so much that before I entered a room, my children would shout, "Mommy's coming!" I loved this, but it irritated Dogbiscuit so I had to return them. The bangles, not the kids.

I tried to gain some affection from Dogbiscuit with my cooking. The way to a man's heart is through his stomach, right? Not if his stomach is bloated with gas, from your food. So I took courses in Italian cuisine, Thai food, and French pastry making. I wasn't terrible. Most of what I made was delicious, but Dogbiscuit wouldn't try anything. Occasionally he'd have a pinch of a chocolate croisant, or bite of a spring roll. For the most part, however, my parents, Dakota, Kate, and Sabatino my stylist, ate the creations I slaved over.

When Dakota noticed how ugly my hands had become from working in the kitchen and sun damaged from pushing the baby carriage, she booked a year of weekly manicures for me. This was one of the nicest things she ever did for me. It also gave me another idea. I signed myself up for massage classes. It was a series of workshops designed for couples. I invited Dogbiscuit to come with me. He practically slapped me in the face. "I don't need massages, I need money," he barked. He was upset with me because he was the one who had to foot the bill for my clothes, and my courses. I'd finished my degree by going to night school, but I didn't work. I stayed at home with our children during the day, and in the evenings I took courses. I decided right then and there that we needed a nanny so I could get a job and become financially responsible for myself.

Dogbiscuit didn't agree, immediately. I had to work him over with the idea that he'd never have to spend another dime on me. Not even at Christmas time. This pleased him to no end. In the fall, when Mackenzie entered grade one and Connor was in kindergarten, we hired Margaret. She became our full-time nanny so I could work part-time.

When I began working at Jason Daniels, a public relations firm, I mistakenly thought Dogbiscuit and I would somehow become closer. We'd have work stories to share with each other over dinner, and we'd want to spend time with the children after being away from them all day. In my mind, I created happy images of us doing things together like a Norman Rockwell painting.

What actually happened was I'd arrive home and take over from Margaret. Dogbiscuit would arrive an hour or so later, fix himself something to eat, and then retire to his den. Sometimes he played with the kids, sometimes he didn't. Usually, I had to look after the baths and bedtime stories. At no time did Dogbiscuit ever inquire about my day, or ask me how I was doing. Once, after a difficult day at the office, I tried to share some of my frustrations with Dogbiscuit. He cut me off with a curt, "You wanted to work. Now take your lumps and live with them."

I never mentioned another thing to him after that. I talked to him about the children, but kept my personal affairs to myself.

I lived with Dogbiscuit in much the same way I lived with Gavin. It wasn't hard to keep things from him, because he had no real interest in what I was doing or what I wanted to do. I filled my life with the small pleasures I gained from working, and the great joys my kids gave me. I wish I could say it was enough, but it wasn't. I had a deep yearning for more. I wanted to feel love and be loved. I craved a warm embrace. It had been years since I'd been kissed by a man, and I couldn't stop myself from wondering how it would feel.

The more I thought about what Dakota had said, the more I realized I did want more out of life. Oh, I didn't want to hurt my family, not even Dogbiscuit. I couldn't be angry with him because he couldn't love me. I don't know what he had planned for his life, but I wasn't it. I couldn't sit idle, oscillating between feeling sorry for Dogbiscuit and sorry for myself.

I looked at the newspaper clipping again. I did want to take a chance on finding a small bit of happiness, even if it meant borrowing someone else's husband. I know this sounds terrible, but a married man who's living the same lie I am, would be able to relate to all the horrors of my life. A single guy might not understand why I continued to stay in a loveless marriage. Most days I didn't know. A married man would understand the sense of commitment that chains you to a person you don't love and who doesn't love you. Only married people really understand when you say, I have to stay for the sake of the kids.

I know this will sound twisted, but in my situation an affair is the only decent thing to do. I can't live without companionship, and sex. I tried and it's making me crazy. I just want a temporary escape that will help me weather the next fifteen to twenty years. If my dream can be fulfilled through a website, who am I to question it? I'll take a chance on what is essentially dot.com hope. It's more than I have now.

"I don't know if you're going to find Prince Charming at Ashley

Madison," Dakota said, trying to keep me grounded, "but you might find someone you can at least talk to."

"That's more than I have right now. I'll take it."

"Yeeeeah!" Dakota actually held up her hands and cheered. A couple of men from the bar looked over at us and smiled. I raised my glass and the cute lawyer-type held up his glass and mouthed the word, "Cheers." Dakota looked over her shoulder quickly, then returned her gaze to me. I guess he wasn't cute enough for her.

"I knew you'd do it. You won't be sorry! This is going to change our lives."

"Our lives?" I said, practically choking on my martini.

"Uhuh." Dakota's mouth was full of her drink. She swallowed and said, "I'm doing it too." I gave her a look, but more on that later.

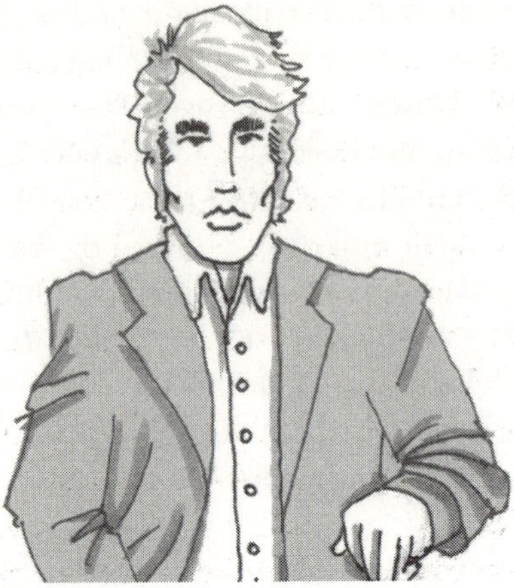

Chapter Two:
The Gentle Man

We left Sassafras around 11:30 and walked over to Dakota's swank apartment on Avenue Road, just north of Bloor Street. We were both very drunk and giddy about the promise of our new adventure. We entered Dakota's building holding hands to help each other remain upright. The concierge gave us a wink like he knew what we were up to. We took the elevator to the ninth floor and when we got off, we headed in opposite directions. This always happens because I get disoriented in Dakota's building. I had to run down the hall to catch up with her. Ironically, she unlocked her door easily, without all the characteristic fumbling she usually does when she's sober.

I headed straight for the den where Dakota kept her computer. Her screen saver was a burst of firecrackers. I sat down on the gorgeous, black, executive office chair in front of her Dell computer. The chair had a cane back, molded arms, and a leather seat. Everything on it moved so it could adjust to the user's body perfectly. The only thing missing was a vibrator for back massages. I had to use my feet to move from one end of the built-in desk to the other. Naturally I minimized my horizontal movements, preferring to swivel myself left, then right. I swiveled very slowly. I didn't want to shake up the martinis sitting happily in my stomach.

I logged onto the Internet and when the computer beeps and groans started, I got up and danced. Dakota came in and danced with me. She brought a bottle of white wine and two glasses. When the computer connected and the beeping stopped, I sat down and typed in Ashleymadison.com. The web page came up and Dakota and I started high-fiving each other as if we'd invented the website ourselves.

"Let's have a drink to celebrate," Dakota said, and we clinked our glasses together. "Here's to Ashley," I said, "a married girl's best friend."

"An attached girl's best friend," Dakota amended.

"Right," I said. I had forgotten about Kalvin. Dakota was living with her boyfriend of six months. His name was Kalvin, with a K, which I hate. It's like Jeff spelled Geoff and Steven with a ph. Entirely unnatural. Like people born with an extra finger, or middle toes that never separated. Kalvin was platinum blond with dark brown eyes and no eyebrows. He was a personal trainer, which meant he was homeless and unemployed. But his abs and biceps were the kind that grace the front cover of *Men's Fitness*.

"Would you really cheat on Kalvin?" I asked Dakota.

"I dunno'. I'm just curious to see what else is out there."

Dakota didn't fool me for a minute. She was frustrated by Kalvin's lack of initiative; that is, his lack of money. Kalvin didn't have any drive and he couldn't make any real plans to do anything because he had no capital to back potential ventures. The Kato Kailin gig was up. The problem was, Dakota wanted him out of her apartment, but not out of her life. I remember her saying something about how handy he was to have around. By that I don't mean anything sexual, although to hear Dakota tell it, Kalvin was such an expert in the bedroom, she had to be peeled off the walls after they made love. Literally. I think Dakota had said that Kalvin was good with power tools and wood. No pun intended. Anyway, if Dakota wanted to hang onto him while she cruised around looking to trade up, who was I to judge?

"Where is Kal?" I asked.

"Bedroom, sleeping," Dakota put her finger over her mouth as if to shush me, but then she banged the wine bottle down loudly, and made noises with her chair and a paper weight. We both laughed.

"You should just tell him to get a real job or leave," I said, turning back to the screen.

"Agreed," Dakota pulled up her leather recliner and I scooted my chair to the left to make room for her. We could both see the computer screen, but we took turns typing, since we were opening two separate accounts. I took out a guest membership, and made Dakota look away while I typed in my password. We had to create profiles of ourselves, stating what we were looking for (tall, dark and handsome), what we were into (shopping, booze, preferably cocktails, and sex not necessarily in that order), what we were hoping to find (bliss). There was space for pictures, however we decided not to post any. We agreed it would add to our intrigue. That, and we weren't computer literate enough to figure out how to get our images uploaded and in the right file.

As an on-screen identity, I used my real first name, Sharon, but added the surname 'Sharalike.' Dakota called herself 'Ecstasy.' She originally wanted Sugarbee, but that was taken. So was Sugar1, Sugar2, Sugar 1970, *Sugar, Brown Sugar, White Sugar, Sugar Girl and Sweet Sugar.

"Maybe I should've picked salt," Dakota said.

"Basil's nice. So is Sage, Parsley, and Thyme," I said, taking a sip of my wine. Dakota stuck her tongue out at me.

"Don't worry about it. What's in a name?" I said, "The men on this site aren't interested in the nickname we give ourselves, they're interested in what we look like, and what we want to do."

"You're nuts. The men on this site are interested in two things: Who wants to fuck them, and where they can meet."

"Do you think?"

"Yeah. Believe me, they aren't looking for stimulating conversation. The last thing they want to do is talk."

"You've never been married, so you don't know how lonely married life can be. I bet a lot of men on this site are looking for a friend."

Dakota started to laugh. "The only friend men want is the kind they can fuck."

"That's not true," I argued. "What about men friends?"

"Them too," she answered. "They want to fuck their women friends in bed, and their men friends in business."

I couldn't argue with her logic, so I poured myself some more wine. We cruised through some of the male profiles, searching the ones with photos, because Dakota didn't trust men who didn't post pictures.

"Well, we didn't post our photos and we're honest and totally trustworthy," I said, pushing my chair back to look at her face.

"Men are far more likely to lie than women."

"Do you think so?"

"Sure. For instance, what are your major fibs?"

"My age and my weight."

"Me too. But men, those bastards, they lie about everything." I couldn't help but think of Kalvin. Having settled on the fact that most men were not trustworthy, we decided not to respond to anyone's ad. We'd wait for men to approach us. Then we would know for sure that they were sincerely interested, not just returning a message the way celebrities respond to fan mail.

Dakota took this one step further and declared she wasn't going to respond to winks. Winks are used to tell someone you're interested. If the recipient is interested, they wink back. The wink sender then sends a message. I liked this feature because it saved time and money. Dakota didn't agree.

"If a guy can't shell out the tokens to send a proper message, he isn't truly interested in you. He's just fishing."

"Anyone who sends a wink to me is going to get a wink back," I declared magnanimously. With all the drinking, I think I might have said rink.

"We'll see about that," Dakota said dubiously.

"I'm going to be really nice. I know what rejection feels like. So I'm going to be really sweet to everyone." I was becoming very emotional, or at least the booze was.

"You don't have a clue about rejection. You married that nutbar a week after your first date."

"Yes, well," I noticed my glass was empty and Dakota was clutching the wine bottle as if it was an Oscar and she was Julia Roberts. I held my glass out to her, and she filled it so full, the wine flowed over my hands, and onto the wool carpet.

"Oops," she said laughing, "I have no depth perception at night." Right.

Once the bottle of Gewürztraminer was finished, the time for my departure had come. Dakota called the concierge, who ordered a cab and buzzed us when it arrived. I had to pour myself into the back seat. I managed to stay upright long enough to wave goodbye to Dakota. Then I pretended I was looking for my earring just so I had an excuse to sprawl across the seat. Thankfully, the cabbie didn't notice I was on my back with my hand across my forehead. Not exactly the kind of position one assumes when trying to locate a missing object.

The fifteen-minute ride to my house was over too soon. When I sat up to pay the cabbie, I realized I'd left my purse at Dakota's. This made me laugh, but the cab driver didn't look amused. His thick eyebrows crinkled up in an angry scowl, which made him look a lot like Osama Bin Ladin.

"No worries," I leaned forward to reassure him, "I'll just pop into the house and get some money. Be right back."

I got out of the car in a crumpled heap. I had to make my way around to the backyard where we keep our spare house key. Dogbiscuit keeps the key under the hat of a hideous looking garden troll, whose eyes, I swear, I've seen move. I had to tromp through wet grass. Dogbiscuit watered the lawn every night. He only had to flick a switch because we had one of those built-in sprinkler systems. But he made as big a deal about it, as if he was actually out there hosing down every last square foot of lawn.

I found the troll okay. The backyard was lit up like a football stadium by all the motion detector lights in ours, and the neighboring yards. The troll's hat was tricky, because it had a rusted latch. I wasn't going to risk breaking a nail, so it took me a while to unhook it. By that time, our neighbor's lights had gone out and things were dim. I finally managed to pry off the troll's hat, and then I had to stick my finger into its haunted, hollow head. All I could see was black. I was sure it was filled with those disgusting, brown, garden beetles, or worse, spiders. I felt like I was on *Fear Factor.* Well I could do this without Joe Rogan's doubting smirk, and false words of encouragement. He only wanted the double-D chicks to win, as if big breasts make the difference between fear and courage. Although, now that I think about it, getting implants that size does require a fair amount of courage. I had that sort of courage, I just wasn't sure how to approach Dogbiscuit for the down payment required to transform my B-cup breasts to a crowd parting, gasp inducing, rack of my own.

I had to use all my courage to fish the spare key out of the troll's head. I took a deep breath and poked around with one finger until I hit metal. I grabbed the key and shut the troll's head. I had made it! I stuck my tongue out at an imagined Joe, then let myself into the house.

I stepped into our family room and kicked my Franko Sarato mules off. All was silent, until I crashed into something that sent searing pain up my shin.

"Christ almighty!" I clamped my mouth shut and put my right hand over my lips, afraid I might wake Dogbiscuit.

I limped to the kitchen where we kept money in a cookie jar for Margaret. Whenever the kids wanted anything, she took money out of the jar. I'm sure she was using the cookie jar to supplement the salary we paid her. Dogbiscuit, for all his financial savvy, hadn't yet realized popsicles and ice cream don't usually cost $64 a week. That's a lot of money for frozen treats. I was this close to pouring Crystal Light into the ice tray, and nixing the cookie jar fund all together. But on a night like this, it sure came in handy. I grabbed a twenty from the jar and hobbled to the front door. I paid the taxi driver and left him a good tip. His face relaxed into a friendly smile, making him look like less like an angry Bin Ladin and more like a Muslim member of ZZ Top.

The next day, I didn't get out of bed until I heard Dogbiscuit leave for work. My head was woozy and my ears felt like they were filled with cotton. So I peed and went back to bed. When I next woke up, I could hear the children leaving the house with Margaret. I got up and went into my daughter's room, which faces the street. A Juliet balcony takes up much of the wall opposite the door. I brushed aside pink shears and unlocked the door so I could yell out to Margaret. She'd already crossed the road with the wagon, sandbox toys and a knapsack.

"Margaret," I shouted, and waited for a sign that she'd heard me. Thankfully, she looked over her shoulder up at me, even as her feet led my children away.

"Where are you off to?" I hollered cupping one hand against the side of my mouth.

Her voice didn't carry well, but it sounded like "park". I closed the door and then it occurred to me that she might very well have said "fuck off". I went back to bed. The phone woke me.

"Hello?"

"Who is this?" It was Dakota. Had the idiot forgotten what number she called?

"It's me, Sharon."

"What's the matter with your voice? You're not sick are you?"

"I'm fine. I've been sleeping," I said, trying to get my voice to sound normal.

"You should get up and log on. I've been at it since 8:30."

I rolled my head so I could see the digital clock, it looked like 10:32, but I wasn't sure. My contacts were blurry.

"Did you get messages already?" I asked her.

"Yes, a couple of winks too, which I didn't respond to."

"Your loss," I half said, half yawned.

"I don't think so. But you'll be losing out if you don't get up soon."

"The messages will still be there when I log on."

"Sure, but there are men who're at work right now, and they have time to do that live instant message thing."

"Really?"

"Yes. Oh, my God, Sharon, I was like, having the ultimate three-way."

"Did you see pictures of these guys?"

"Yes, and they are sooo hot."

"All of them?"

"Two out of three. One is so smoking he makes my mouth water."

"Really?"

"Uh-oh, Kal's back. I gotta' run."

"Where's he been?"

"I sent him on some errands, so I could get on the computer without him trying to rub my shoulders or use his caliper on my thigh muscles."

"Why is he always trying to measure you?"

"I dunno, I think he wants me to hire him as my personal trainer."

"Free room and board isn't enough?"

"You'd think. Some men don't know when they've got a good thing going."

"Yes, men like Dogbiscuit," I said.

"You know, one day he's going to take his head out of his ass, and when he does, he'll not only be filled with regret, but also remorse for the way he's treated you."

"I'm not sure that's ever going to happen."

"Trust me, it will. However, by then, you will have moved on to someone who can appreciate how fabulous you are."

On that positive note, I said goodbye. It was anyone's guess why Dogbiscuit preferred his friends, his work as an investment banker, and his lawn, to me. My efforts to transform myself into Housewife of the Year, have largely been met with indifference, if not down right hostility. I'm not just referring to the massage course (which, by the way, I attended without a partner). The instructor was kind enough to allow me to practice on him, and occasionally when someone's spouse was absent, I had a different partner. Altogether, it wasn't a bad experience, but the only one who benefits from what I learned is my son Connor. Mackenzie finds the kneading of her flesh bothersome, and Dogbiscuit refuses to allow me anywhere near his body.

I've been enduring this uncomfortable state of marital agony since before Connor was born. Indeed, the conception of my son is somewhat of a mystery to me. I honestly can't remember doing the mambo in bed sheets with Dogbiscuit. We lived like two roommates who could barely tolerate each other.

He has his life, his work, and his friends, most of whom don't like me even though they've met me only once or twice. Whatever Dogbiscuit told them about me, was enough for them to keep me at arms-length.

The only time Dogbiscuit takes an interest in me is when I'm indulging in self-depreciating humor. I used to do it quite a lot, despite the fact that Kate and Dakota thought it was a form of self-hate. When I put myself down, it made Dogbiscuit laugh and he would join in with a gusto that would've made Joan Rivers cringe. I gave up the self-depreciating remarks when I heard Mackenzie doing the same. She was now in the third grade, and her self-image was being formed, not only by what I told her about herself, but also by the way she perceived me. It broke my heart to hear her call herself stupid. Once she even asked Connor if she looked fat in her leotards.

I put an end to the nasty remarks about myself, even though it seemed to drive Dogbiscuit farther away from me. If I had to choose between him and my children, there was no contest. I wanted to be the best mother I could be. For me, that meant not only doing motherly things, like making mud pies in the backyard, but looking good while doing them. I worked hard to emulate the familial happiness of the Calvin Klein ads featuring Christy Turlington with some gorgeous guy pretending to be her husband and a young model playing the role of their laughing child. I had to do this without Dogbiscuit, which suited me. He isn't very good at being happily married, or gorgeous. More importantly however, neither Mackenzie nor Connor seemed to miss him. In fact, our threesome seemed natural.

I devoted myself to my children and my appearance. I wasn't a fashion junkie, but I was close. Maybe too close. For the most part I ignored Dogbiscuit's scowls, groans, and insulting remarks. If he wasn't willing to acknowledge that his wife was a cross between Pamela Anderson and Martha Stewart, it was his loss. What seemed to make Dogbiscuit feel better about himself, was telling me how awful I looked. Just this morning, he woke me up to tell me my eyes looked bloodshot. Remembering this, I rolled over and made a grab for the make-up mirror in the end table. Ooh, I did indeed look dreadful. I should've put a paper bag over my head instead of just an eye mask. I was suffering the effects of too much liquor and not enough food. It's a temporary condition, which can be remedied by Champagne and orange juice. Bacon and eggs wouldn't hurt either.

I got out of bed and headed for the shower. Unlike Dakota, I have to go to work to collect a regular paycheck. Dakota is a flight attendant with Air Canada. She works eight days a month non-stop, then hibernates for three days after her last shift ends. This month, she has returns to Jamaica, which she loves. Dakota comes from a wealthy family who made their money through hard work and wise investments. She doesn't actually have to work; she has a trust fund she can draw from. When we were in university, her grandmother died and left her an enormous amount of money. I asked her how much, but she never told me. I know it has to be more than a million. After she graduated with her Bachelor's degree, she hung out in Italy for about two years. She sent really cute wooden toys for Mackenzie, and leather for me. At the time, she was dating a photographer. He took some really stunning photographs of her, which she also sent to me.

When that relationship soured, she came home.

During her very first visit to my house, she witnessed my unhappiness. I'd kept much of it from her by talking about Mackenzie whenever we spoke on the phone. However, when she saw me in person, I couldn't hide the truth from her. With the memory of her own defunct relationship fresh in her mind, she tried to persuade me to leave Dogbiscuit, but I didn't. She kept telling me I could set myself up in a downtown condo, but I just didn't want to do the single mother thing. Little did I know I'd end up living like a single mom anyway, since it was just easier than having to deal with Dogbiscuit.

Dakota was the one who bought the condo. We spent hours shopping for just the right furnishings and accessories. It was so much fun, I wished I had purchased a place of my own. Whenever I tried to bring anything into the house that Dogbiscuit bought, I ended up returning it. His criticisms were so severe, it just wasn't worth the battle. The only rooms I decorated were those of my children. Dogbiscuit and his mother looked after the rest. That's how I ended up with a chintz covered couch with rolled arms, instead of a tuxedo couch in chocolate leather. Ironically, after putting her decorating stamp in almost every room of the house, Dogbiscuit's mother rarely came to visit. He went to her house in Lawrence Park.

Dakota wanted me to become a flight attendant. I was going to do it, because I'm fluent in French, but I didn't. A job like that would require me to be away from home too much, and the problem with that was I might actually like it. This wouldn't be good for my kids. If they had to have Dogbiscuit for a dad, the least I could do was stick around for them.

My job isn't anywhere near as glamorous as Dakota's, but at least I have regular hours as a part-time copy editor. I'm home in the mornings and again at night. Margaret looks after the children in the hours between.

I like my job, but I find the noon to six shift a bit tough. Just as I settle into beginning my working day, my stomach starts to growl for lunch. Everyone says eat before you start, but do you think that helps? No. Psychologically, my body starts to crave food on the hour, every hour from noon to two o'clock, and I don't get a break until three.

I arrived at work just before noon that day. The office is always a beehive of activity in the morning, but at noon, people start taking their lunch breaks and things quiet down until 3:30, when the pace picks up again. I have a small, windowless cubicle, like most of the other staff. My only consolation is the great computer I was given. It even has a high-speed Internet connection. I know that for lots of people that's a standard feature, but you have no idea of the primitive conditions I work under. As soon as I sat down, I logged onto the Ashley Madison website. I typed in my password and found seven messages waiting for me.

I have to admit, this was starting to titillate me. The notion of sitting back while a bevy of men vied for my attention was quite the turn-on. I felt like a kid in a candy store. Even better, a kid in a candy store with free samples, who could try all the candy she wanted.

Two guys who contacted me sounded like they were looking for sex and only sex, so I deleted their messages. One guy had a mustache, which I'm not into, so I sent a nice message to him basically saying, *Thanks, but no thanks*. The other four all sounded good, and looked even better. Three of them had pictures posted with their profile. The one without a picture called himself Gentle Man. His age was forty, which of course meant he was older. His height was a perfect six-foot-two and his weight was an ideal 185 pounds. Right! In his profile, he said he wanted to meet a special girl to create an experience unlike any he'd ever had before. That sounded like a tall order to me. Then I read the part that said he wanted a girl to pamper. After that, I was thinking, why settle for an affair? Hell, let's get married and then you can pamper me twenty-four-seven. When I hear the word pamper, I think of days spent at Clear Water Spa and dinners at Morton's.

Gentle Man went on to say he enjoyed holding hands, walking in the rain, watching movies, playing basketball, and dining in fine restaurants. I know that sounds a bit like an old Barry Manilow song, but who cares? If this guy was even halfway cute, I'd be up for at least one date. I crossed my fingers. He said he'd exchange pictures with any interested lady.

His private message to me was, *Cinnamon twist* (How cute is that?) *you sound sweet, I think we should meet*. (I do too!) *Holler back if you're interested, lady*.

I was so interested! I sent back a message that said, *Gentle man, I think I am the gentle woman you seek. Send me your pic and then we shall meet*.

I wasn't really intending to rhyme, it just happened. I hope he doesn't send back another rhyme because that can become tiresome. I had to log off the Ashley Madison site because sooner or later, someone was going to dip his or her head over the partition to say hi to me, or order me to do something, like work. My day was uneventful, and as I got up to leave at 5:45, I remembered Ashley. So I sat back down and restarted my computer.

"Sharon, working late?"

I looked up at Ralph, feeling like a cat caught with budgie feathers in its mouth. Ralph is first assistant to one of the firm's junior directors. In short, this means he's a gofer. He thinks his job is more important than mine because he sometimes arrives at my desk bearing messages like, "I need your attention on this ASAP" or "This has to be done *now*," or the one I hate, "Bill won't accept this. You need to redo it." The worst part about Ralph is that he knows everything. Not in a universal sense, but he knows all the goings and comings of our office. When a new high-profile contract comes in, Ralph will know all the details. If someone is about to be pink slipped, Ralph will have that information too. I liked him, but I knew I had to be careful, because a word from Ralph into the right ear, could result in terrible repercussions. If you were having a party and you wanted everyone in the office to attend, you didn't have to bother with invitations. All one had to do was inform Ralph, and everyone would know.

"No," I said to Ralph. Then I caught myself and added rather clumsily, "I mean yes. I'm trying to stay on top of things."

"Really? That's so unlike you."

"I'm turning over a new leaf," I said, glad that Ralph couldn't see my screen from where he was. I'd already clicked on the address for Ashley Madison, any second it would come up and I'd be caught.

"Well, if you'll excuse me."

"Sure, carry on," he said. I expected Ralph to push off, but he didn't move. I got out a manila folder and started rummaging through it as if I was looking for something important.

Ralph moved off just as the website came up. I typed in my password, then reduced the screen size. I stood up and scanned the office. There were two people in payroll. No one else was around. I sat down again, enlarged the screen and found a message from Gentle Man waiting for me. He'd sent a key I could use to view his pictures, and best of all, he left this message:

If you like what you see, call me. And he sent his phone number.

I clicked on the key. Three pictures came up. Wow, he was so fantastic looking. I could sum him up in three simple words: finger licking good. The first picture showed off rippling muscles, a washboard stomach, and a treasure trail that disappeared inside the waistband of his faded jeans. The second picture was taken in a gym. His arms and chest looked like they were about to explode. He was clearly a slave to his body. In the third picture, Gentle Man was dressed in a tuxedo. He looked like he was in a wedding party, his own perhaps. A touch of gray around his temples gave him that really distinguished look. I picked up my phone to call him, and punched the digits in very slowly so I wouldn't make a mistake. By the time I got to the last digit, my heart was beating so loudly I could hear it. To calm myself down, I took a deep breath and decided to count to thirty before I hung up. I got to three. He answered on the first ring,

"Mike," came the no-nonsense greeting.

"Hello, Mike?"

"Yup, who's calling?"

"Cinnamon twist," I said, smiling into the phone. Oh God, what if I wasn't the only woman he'd nicknamed that? I was so nervous, my hand was shaking. Sweat was pouring off me like rain.

"Hey sweetie, how are you?"

"I'm good, thanks." That sounded too formal. I'd better fun it up, or he'll think I'm an uptight wife.

"I didn't expect you to respond so quickly. You must have liked those pictures," he laughed. I laughed too.

"They were nice. Thanks for letting me see them."

"Not a problem. When do I get to see you?"

"You know what?" I wasn't expecting him to answer me, but he *did*.

"No, what?"

"I don't have any pictures."

"Hon, I don't want to see pictures."

"You don't?"

"No doll, I want to see you," he said. This was followed by the sexiest chuckle ever.

"Um, well, okay."

"You sound uncertain. Do you want to think about it and get back to me?"

"No, no. I'd like to meet you too. I'm just nervous. I've never done anything like this before." I dried my hands on my skirt.

"I haven't either, but I've spent so much time thinking about doing it, that the reality of it feels pretty close to what I imagined." That made me wonder if I should have thought this through. Could I really go through with it?

"How do you want to proceed?" Mike asked, breaking into my thoughts.

"I don't know," I confessed.

"Would you like to meet me? I'd love to meet you."

"Okay," I said. I was so flattered.

"Great, let's meet for lunch tomorrow, say around one o'clock."

"Okay, where?" Why did I agree to that time? I can't meet him at one o'clock. I have to work!

"In what part of the city are you located?" he asked. I know he was only following simple, get-together protocol, but I suddenly felt a relentless, Terminator-style pursuit closing in on me.

"I'm central. I can get anywhere," I answered, in spite of my growing fear.

"Good girl, I like that." Oh my God, this guy was making my pulse beat so fast, I was going to have a heart attack.

"Where would you like to meet?" I asked, trying to keep the oxygen flowing into my lungs.

"Can you get to the Sutton Place Hotel?"

A hotel? Already? I don't even know this guy.

"You want to meet at a hotel?"

"Doll, relax. We're having lunch. That's it. I don't even know what you look like." Again the sexy laugh. Extra sexy this time.

"Right," I said breathing a sigh of relief.

"What are you going to be wearing?" Oh my God. I hadn't thought that far. I've done zero shopping for this. I could get to the mall after dinner, but that didn't help me now. What should I tell Mike I'd be wearing? Think, think, think.

"Black skirt," I blurted out.

"Will you be wearing anything else with that?"

"Yes," I said laughing.

"You don't have to. I read your profile and with measurements like that, you probably look outstanding with nothing on."

Could this guy be any more charming? I was speechless for a moment, then I recovered enough to say,"I don't know what top I'll be wearing, but my skirt is short, and I'll have boots on."

"The kind with heels?"

"Yes," I said, amazed that he'd even think to ask.

"I love that look." Me too.

"Okay," I said, "so you'll be able to spot me?"

"I'll do my best."

"See you tomorrow," I said, already moving the earpiece away from my face.

"One o'clock, Sutton Place Hotel."

I moved the earpiece back.

"Right." I confirmed, even though I still didn't know how I was going to swing it.

"Is there a number I can reach you at if there's a problem?"

"Sure," I said. I gave him my cell number and said goodbye. I started to return the phone to the cradle.

"Cinnamon?"

"Yes?" I brought the phone back to my ear yet again.

"What's your real name?"

"Sharon."

"Really?" he sounded incredulous.

"Yeah."

"You know what, Sharon?"

"What?"

"I think I'm in love." We both laughed. Then I hung up, and I thought that was the hottest, sweatiest conversation I'd had in a long time. Imagine what phone sex would be like.

The next morning, I called in sick. When Margaret left with the kids, I started to get ready. I didn't have time to go to the mall, so I had to wear something I already owned. I flung all sorts of clothes out of my closet and onto the bed. I tried on at least a dozen different sweaters, blouses, and shirts. Finally, I settled on a geometric print top with a black and cream pattern. It looked very sixties chic with the black mini and knee-high boots. I put on a black bolero jacket, since the weather was a bit cool. I put my hair into one of those high ponytails. I looked like the next Austin Powers sex kitten.

I met Mike at the bar in the lobby of the Sutton Place Hotel. I was ten minutes late, but he didn't seem to mind. He got up as soon as I walked in and held out his hand to take mine. He pulled me in for a hug. He smelled like lemon and cedar. Mike was tall and handsome in a Pierce Brosnan kind of way. He was definitely older than forty but his body looked like it belonged to a twenty-five-year-old. I couldn't stop smiling all through lunch. He was so much fun to be with. He was funny, he wasn't too old, he had great teeth, and he liked me. He really liked me.

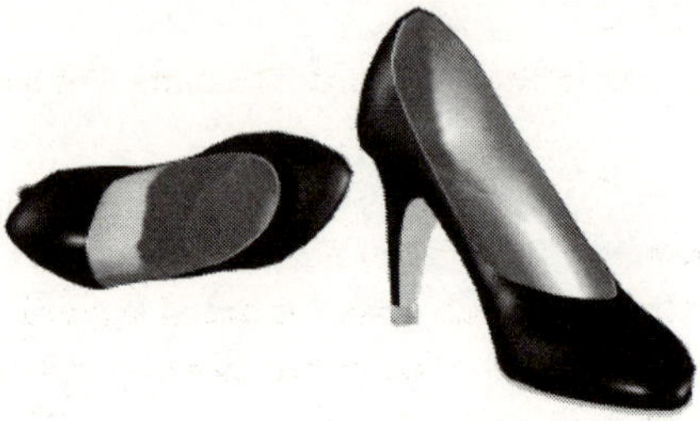

Chapter Three:
Dinky Dick

Okay, now I was sure Mike liked me, because he actually said so. During our lunch date at the hotel, he said, "Sharon, you're very pretty, and I'm stunned your husband doesn't have you on a pedestal." He actually said stunned, and when he said the word, his eyes closed for a second, like he was trying to remove from his mind the unimaginable thought of a man not putting a wife like me on a pedestal. I found myself nodding at Mike in agreement. "You're a gorgeous young woman, and if you were my wife, I'd treat you like a queen."

"Really?"

"Absolutely," he sounded emphatic.

"Is that how you treat your wife?"

"More or less. She thinks I'm an ATM machine, so it's never occurred to her to show an ounce of gratitude or a measure of appreciation."

"That's really terrible. Is that why you're looking for...?" I let my voice trail off. I didn't know how to finish my sentence. What was he looking for? A girlfriend? A replacement for his wife? A mistress?

Mike, sensing my uncertainty said, "I'm looking for someone I can get close to without worrying how much it's going to cost me." That made me laugh, but Mike's face was serious.

"Sorry," I apologized, but I was grinning madly.

"It's okay," he said leaning forward. "Either you laugh or you cry, right?"

"So true," I said.

Then Mike caught me off guard by asking, "What are you looking for?"

"I'm not sure," I said honestly. I didn't just want a sex partner. I wanted someone I could be with. Someone who would share my two-for-one Dairy Queen coupons. I wanted someone to go with to the movies on Friday night, and roller blading on Sunday morning. I guess what I wanted was a boyfriend. I know I'm too old and too married for that, but truth be told, I needed a stunt double for Dogbiscuit. Just for the record, I prefer the tall, dark-haired, blue-eyed types. Mike looked a lot like what I wanted. He was handsome, he seemed kind, and he was definitely fun to be with. All systems were locked on target.

"I think you might be what I need," I said shyly.

"I'm glad you think so, doll, because you definitely look like the antidote to my ailments." That made me laugh out loud in one of those super model, show all your teeth grins.

"I don't know about that," I said looking down at my lap. It was covered in a white napkin and breadcrumbs. I dusted my napkin off before looking up. When I did, my eyes met Mike's azure gaze. I felt a jolt move right through me, from my stomach to my heart. I looked away and reached for my water glass. Mike moved his arm across the table and brushed his fingers against mine.

"You have beautiful hands," he said. He covered my hand with his own, and as soon as I felt the warmth of his palm, my heart stopped beating. When it started again it was doing double-time, and I was certain Mike could hear it across the small table. I moved my hand away from the glass, and placed it on the table. Mike kept his hand over mine, like he was my shadow.

"Where do we go from here?" he asked.

I was tempted to say tenth floor, south-facing room. Instead I said, "Should we have lunch again next week?"

"We've done lunch. Can you get away for dinner?"

"Sure," I said, as an image of Dogbiscuit's pinched face crossed my mind. He doesn't like it when I'm not home during dinner because he can't manage the kids after Margaret leaves. I'm not much better. I admit I'm no mother of the year, but at least I have a relationship with the kids. When I look at them, I don't just see income tax deductions that need flu shots every year. Dogbiscuit prefers it when I'm with him at dinner so we can tag team to wrestle the kids into the docile kind you see on TV sit-coms. Come to think of it, it's probably the only time he prefers me being with him. Our alliance lasts until they're fed, bathed, and put to bed. We've tried getting Margaret to stay until 7:30, but she complains that her days are long enough already.

"What night is good for you?" Mike's question snapped me back to the situation at hand. And speaking of hands, he was still holding mine. I wanted to take a sip of water, but I couldn't use my left hand because that would have been too awkward, and my right hand was paralyzed under Mike's warm fingers. I liked the feeling of his hand on mine, it was very secure and comforting. It made me feel desirable. I suddenly felt so superior to all the other women in the restaurant. They were probably jealous of me right now.

"Any night is good." Did you hear that ladies? He's asking me which night is good for me. Ha, ha, they're all looking at us… Oh my God! They're all looking at us! I suddenly realized the enormity of what I was doing. I was making a future date with someone clearly not my husband, completely out in the open for the whole world to see.

"Next Thursday?" Mike was still making date arrangments, blithely oblivious that I was having a full-blown panic attack. His hand, still firmly planted on mine, seemed to emanate a siren noise. I tried to stay as composed as possible. I didn't want him to know what I was fretting about.

"Thursday should be... oh wait a minute, I think I might have something on Thursday. What about Friday?" What the hell was I doing? Agree to a future date and get out of there as fast as humanly possible, you ninny.

"That doesn't work for me." He sounded disappointed. I quickly offered, "Wednesday?" I was ready to rattle off every day of the week for the next four months.

"I play hockey with the guys."

Oh for the…"Can't you miss a game?"

"Yes, but I want to keep things as normal as possible if I'm going to be... you know?"

"Yes, of course," I said leaning forward. "I know exactly what you mean. We don't want to call any unnecessary attention to ourselves."

Holding hands in public was probably the last thing we should've been doing. I wasn't about to pull my hand away because it felt so right. I knew it was entirely acceptable for me to be seen at lunch with a man who could've been my boss, or a co-worker, or a potential client. But there was no way this kind of hand holding could be explained away as anything other than what it appeared to be: two lovers, or potential lovers, sharing a moment of intimacy. Knowing this should have made me recoil in caution, but I didn't. I've never held hands with a man other than my father. The experience was far too pleasurable for me to voluntarily bring it to an end.

"To be successful at this game, we should keep our patterns as regular as possible."

"Right, okay. Well, Tuesday won't work for me." I wish it did, oh how I wish it did. At this point, I was ready to gnaw off a limb to get out of whatever previous engagement was keeping me from just saying yes so we could wrap up lunch.

"Monday?" He gave my hand a little squeeze. I wanted to say yes, but Mondays I have a Kick Boxing class I was reluctant to give up. After all, how ironic would it be if Mike was a rapist and I was with him the night I should've been learning the best way to inflict groin injury? I shook my head.

"How about the following week?" I suggested.

"On Thursday?"

"I should be free." I wasn't certain, but at that moment I couldn't think of any up-coming event. As soon as I got home I'd check the kitchen calendar. That's where Margaret, Dogbiscuit and I kept track of household comings and goings and anything related to the children.

"Okay, my fingers are crossed." He actually crossed his fingers on both hands. Could this guy be any cuter? When Mike took his hand off mine, I curled my fingers up and slipped my hand into my lap.

I eyed my water glass up and down. I didn't think I could keep my hand steady enough to raise it to my lips, so I just sat there with a parched throat, wondering how Mike got so cute and so charming in only forty-six years. He told me the truth about his age fifteen minutes after we met. Good thing, because I was going to say something to the effect that he was one old looking forty-year-old. I told him that I'm really thirty-three, and he said I looked twenty-five. You see what I mean about his charm? This guy could run laps around Dogbiscuit.

"My fingers are crossed too," I said even though they weren't. My hands were entwined on my lap.

"I'll call you. Your cell is okay?"

"Yes, it's totally secure." Dogbiscuit would never answer my phone, even if it was sitting on his dinner plate.

"I'll call you," Mike said, with the sincerity of Mother Teresa.

Three weeks later, Mike still hadn't called me. I didn't want to act like a pre-pubescent twelve-year-old juiced up on Justin Timberlake, but I couldn't help myself. I was constantly wondering why hadn't he called. I kept checking my cell phone for messages, but there weren't any from Mike. None. I even called myself a few times to make sure my phone was working. It was. I went to the Ashley Madison website at least half-a-dozen times and never found him signed on. One day, I clicked on his profile and it said he hadn't been on in twelve days. What was up with that? Why the disappearing act? Did he quit and forget to tell me? I wondered if it might be okay to call him? After all, he might have lost my number.

I kept looking at the calendar in the kitchen thinking I should just ring him to make sure I didn't get the date mixed up. I'm sure we agreed to skip a week because our schedules weren't cooperating with our desires. That would mean last Thursday should have been our dinner date. Maybe he thought I was going to call. Maybe he was sitting in his office right now wondering what had happened to me. I should ring him and say something like, I've been thinking of you. That would be the truth too; thinking about why that lying bastard hadn't called me. I picked up the phone and called my cousin Kate.

"Hello?" Kate's voice sounded sleepy. I looked at the kitchen clock. It was 2:15. Dogbiscuit had taken the children to Silver City. They wouldn't be back until after four. I could talk to Kate for a while and then call Mike.

"How long should a girl wait for a guy to call after he's said, 'I'll call you?'"

"Who is this?"

"It's Sharon," I rolled my eyes. How could she not know it was me?

"Who's the guy?"

"Does it matter?"

"Well, of course it matters. If the guy is serious about you, he'll call within two days. If he calls any time after that, you're on the second string."

"Really?"

"Oh yeah, you're a bench warmer honey. You're good for substitutions and that's about it." Since we were talking about a married man, I wasn't offended. I couldn't expect to come first in Mike's life. I just wanted him to call me.

"Okay, so how long does a girl wait for the promised phone call?"

"Don't wait. Call him."

"Won't that seem too desperate?"

"Desperate? Of course not. But on the other hand, you're chained to an albatross who can't supply any sexual healing, so in a way, hon, you are desperate."

"Well, that might be true, but I don't have to wear my misery on my sleeve, do I?"

"No, so when you call him, be really cool and very casual."

"Okay," I said checking the wall clock to make sure I'd have enough time to make the call before Dogbiscuit returned.

"When you get in touch with him, what are you planning to do?"

"I haven't planned anything. I'm the spontaneous type. I'll do whatever I feel like." Geez, was that me talking? I doubt Kate believed me, because even I didn't.

"Mmm-hm, spontaneous huh? Sounds like you're looking for some you-know-what. Kate liked to think she was with it and daring, but saying things like you-know-what made it painfully obvious she wasn't.

"I'm going to wait another day and see if he calls."

"Why, do you think the cast is coming off his dialing finger tomorrow?" That made me giggle.

"I'm sure he's fine, but he could be away on business or something."

"Look, I don't know this guy, and I just woke up when you called, so maybe nothing I'm going to say will make any sense, but the way I see it is, if a guy hasn't called after a week, he isn't going to call. So girlfriend, move on. There are plenty of fish in the sea. Dump that phone phobic loser and cast your line again. I'm sure there are plenty more where you found him, right?"

"Yes, I suppose," I felt so rejected. Mike's never going to call me? How could he sound so sincere? And he said he wanted to go to dinner; was that a lie?

"Why do you sound so sad?" Kate asked.

"I really liked him and I believed him when he said he'd call."

"Men always say that. It's just one of those phrases people use as conversation filler."

"Really?"

"Sure. Like when you say to someone you run into at the mall, 'We should get together.' You don't really mean it, but after you've told her she looks great and you love her shoes, which you wish were yours, what else can you say? 'Let's get together. Call me or I'll call you,' is a nice way to ease into 'Goodbye.' Men use a lot of empty phrases."

I took Kate's advice and spent every free moment of the next week sending and receiving instant messages to at least seventeen different men. Some were real bores, a few were gems, and others were so annoying, I felt absolute pity for their wives. One guy, BorntoPlease insisted I was a man because I hadn't posted my picture. Our conversation went like this:

BorntoPlease: *If you are a woman, show yourself.*

Sharon Sharalike: *I don't have a picture.*

BorntoPlease: *That's because you're a man.*

Sharon Sharalike: *You're an 'A' hole.*

BorntoPlease: *Yes, but you're a man.*

Sharon Sharalike: *Why don't you leave me alone and go fuck your wife?*

BorntoPlease: *I much prefer fucking other people's wives.*

At that point I terminated the conversation by blocking him. He can't send me any more messages unless I unblock him and that's never going to happen.

BorntoPlease is one of those rare exceptions I sometimes came across between noon and four o'clock. I'd started going to work at 11:30 so I could get more time on the Ashley Madison website. Margaret took this as a sign of my maturing.

"It's high time you started taking a serious approach to work."

"Yes," I said. Margaret had a way of reducing me to a contrite ten-year-old.

"When the children are older you can work full-time."

"Right," I said. Work full-time, was she insane? When would I go shopping? How would I schedule my manicures? Already I was feeling the immeasurable strain of working part-time. Any more hours, and my minimal social life would vanish like a cheap magician's trick. The only thing that kept me going to work was high-speed Internet access and the regular paycheck, which kept me in Franco Sarto shoes. Dogbiscuit said if I stopped working, he'd put me on a budget. Can you imagine me at Payless, fighting Star Jones for the last pair of size eight patent leather clogs? I think I'll keep working.

I've learned how to keep the Ashley Madison window open, hidden under three other windows, so when people come near my desk at work, a click of my mouse hides it in seconds. The best part is, I look like I'm engrossed in some serious work. Nobody bothers me and if they do, they deal with me quickly, so I can get on with my work, because I'm obviously a very busy person. I've also started to keep lots of papers strewn about.

Ralph has noticed. Yesterday he said to me, "Sharon you've really got your nose to the grindstone these days, haven't you?"

"Yes, I'm exceptionally busy." I gave him a look that should have stopped time, but he ignored it.

"You're not using office hours to chat with your girlfriends anymore are you?"

"Can you go fuck off now? I'm busy." I said the 'fuck off' in a whisper so I wouldn't get fired.

"Tsk, tsk," he said, without moving.

I started to remove my left shoe and Ralph took off. He was a big fan of Jerry Springer so he knew what it meant when a woman grabbed her throwing shoe. I'm sure he didn't relish the idea of shielding his face from an ankle boot with a two-and-three-quarter inch heel. I've been trying to schedule my lunches at the same time

Ralph has his afternoon coffee break. I do this so he won't have an excuse to skulk around my desk to tell me something stupid when I'm in the middle of instant messaging some hottie.

Speaking of which, I'd found a new potential. Online he called himself Concobar. I recognized that name right away. My son's name, Connor, is derived from Concobar honoring the heroic Irish king. My mother-in-law would probably approve of Concobar because he was hard-core Irish, at least his name was. His first name was Rick, short for Carrick. I didn't think you could get more Irish than that.

Rick and I had been corresponding almost non-stop through e-mails, and messages on MadAsh, what I'd started calling the Ashley Madison website. I'd gotten into the groove of picking up messages in the morning and sending new ones before leaving the office at six. That day, however, I received a message from Rick indicating he wanted to meet online after nine for instant messaging. I wanted to do this, because sending and receiving messages in real time is so much more fun. I couldn't do it at home because I don't have access to the Internet. Dogbiscuit's computer was hooked up, but I wasn't allowed to use it. It was in the den and Dogbiscuit didn't allow me in there; my female hormones might contaminate the male testosterone in the dark chamber. In other words, two years earlier, I'd spilled a bottle of OPI nail polish on the Persian carpet. It was Matador Red, and the best the stain remover could do was reduce it to Cherokee Brown. So now, Dogbiscuit's den looks like the scene of a homicide. All that's missing is the chalky white outline of the slain victim. I've offered to pose for this, but Dogbiscuit refuses. I used to watch a lot of *Colombo*, so I knew how to position my body to make it look like I'd died of a gunshot wound. Believe me, it's come in handy. I've used it on more than one occasion to fake my way out of Dogbiscuit's three-step sex routine, which could be summed up as two tweaks and a poke. Most of the time he didn't even bother, and that was fine by me, but a woman cannot live by vibrator alone. I didn't even have one, so I was desperate to find a stand-in for Dogbiscuit.

I had to find a way to get to the Internet on my laptop at home. During my lunch break I asked Ralph,"Is there a way I could hookup my laptop to another computer with Internet access and piggyback into cyberspace?"

"No," Ralph said, taking a bite of banana bread.

"Is that a 'no, you don't know how', or a 'no, it can't be done?'"

"I don't know how to do it because it can't be done."

"Right. Well then, if I want Internet on my laptop at home, and another computer in the same home already has Internet access, and is actually logged on when I turn on my system."

"How fast will both trains be going if they pass each other at 7:30?"

"Very funny," I said, sarcastically.

"Oh I'm sorry, I thought you were setting up a math problem."

I started to get up, but Ralph stopped me.

"Wait a minute Sharon, where are you going?"

"Back to work," I said.

"Do you have Internet on cable on the first computer?"

"I don't think so," I said.

"You could get that, for your laptop. You could also get another dial-up or you could buy a splitter box and use the same Internet server you've got on the PC."

"Ralph you're the best," I said. I gave him one of those hugs that only involve shoulders.

"I do what I can," he said, taking another bite of banana bread.

"Thank you so much," I said getting up with my Diet Coke and fourteen grapes.

I had started a new, get-fit-for-sex diet, even though I wasn't fat or anything. I just thought five pounds might make the difference between delicious and sex-a-licious. My guess was most men prefer the latter. I figured a little bit of weight loss would lean out my body so I could get the angular Victoria's Secret look without losing all my curves. If I was going into a new relationship, I needed to look fantastic, right? I should give my new guy something to write home about. I needed to add *Cosmopolitan* to my shopping list. There was no sense in having a gorgeous body if I didn't know how to use it.

Dogbiscuit was the only man who'd ever seen me naked. He reluctantly gave me two thumbs-up, probably because two thumbs down required slightly more physical effort. As a result of his indifference, I worried about how another man might rate me. I knew I shouldn't even be thinking that, but after Mike left me at the alter, so to speak, I felt like maybe I wasn't so hot. You know? I mean nowadays, women have to compete with sexy teens and twenty-somethings in music videos. And then there are the cuter than thou models in women's magazines. Just when I started becoming immune to the beauty of super models, men's magazines raised the bar a notch higher. Have you seen the latest *Maxim* covers? I was so tired of all those cellulite-free, flat-bellied, long-legged, scantily clad, double-D, silicone chicks. Yes, Carmen Electra, I am talking about you.

It's not that I was jealous or anything. I knew stunning beauty required pain, sacrifice, and discipline. (Read: waxing, no female friends for shopping, stalkers, and a reduced calorie, low-carb diet). I just wanted to know why I couldn't enjoy the benefits of airbrushing every time I stepped into the real world, wearing only a micro-bikini and a smile.

After my lunch break, I sent Rick an e-mail explaining that I couldn't meet him online that evening. It would take me a couple of days to find an Internet service provider and get things set up at home. I had to hope Dogbiscuit wouldn't ask any questions. At such times, his nose started twitching like the Shaggy D.A. looking for clues.

When I got home from work, my daughter displayed an uncharacteristic interest in me. Margaret must have disciplined her about something. Now I was Mackenzie's best friend. That actually suited me because it had been ages since I'd had a chance to play with Fashion Polly Pocket and her crew. My daughter had at least six different Fashion Polly dolls.What bugged me about the Polly Pocket collectibles, was that for all those girl dolls, there was only one boy doll, a surfer dude who wears his name, Rick, across his chest. All the girls had to compete for this toy-boy's affections, not unlike life in the real world. Good men are so scarce, the odds of finding a nice looking, employed, straight, monogamous, (Oops! Cancel monogamous and substitute rich) romantic guy, is about one in four. With those odds, many women were going to have to learn to share. Polly and her pals didn't seem to mind. And you should see the look on Rick's face. He smiles twenty-four-seven. Never mind that his grin is painted on.

While we were playing, Mackenzie insisted on listening to a Sharon, Lois, and Bram CD. Mackenzie and I played and sang until dinner. After dinner, Mackenzie continued to delight in my company, so we had a wonderful bath-time experience with bubbles, giggles and hugs. As I watched her pile bubbles over her chubby body, it occured to me that raising my children should be enough. The joy I felt at that moment was bliss. Yet it failed to sustain me. When I thought about how I was going to spend the rest of my evening and the rest of my life, I knew I could never be happy just being a mother. I needed something for me too.

When nine o'clock rolled around, my heart sank because Rick would be logging on, expecting to chat with me and instead, he'd find my cold and empty message. I must have sighed loudly because Dogbiscuit lowered his newspaper and fixed me with a scowl so nasty, it made me want to put up my fists. Instead, I slipped out of the house and went for a run.

The next morning, I arrived at work at 11:15, my earliest time ever. It was weird being in the office so early. The vibe was completely different. Everyone walked around bleary eyed, talking about last night's television shows. I never watch TV, so I didn't have a clue what they were talking about. Just as well; I didn't come in early to chitchat. I was there to check my messages on MadAsh.

I was exchanging messages on a daily basis with Rick and about five other guys. Although Rick was my favorite, I'd learned the hard way from Mike not to put all my eggs in one basket. I really wanted things to work out with Rick, but if they didn't, at least I could move to plan B. At this moment plan B was shaping up to be an entrepreneur with a startling resemblance to Alec Baldwin. For the first time in my life, I felt like I was in a win-win situation.

Rick's message to me was so filled with longing, it made me want to pick up the phone and call him. Unfortunately, I didn't have his number and he never asked for mine. So I sent him my cell number with only two words written in my message: *Call me*. At eleven minutes after three, my cell phone rang. Guess who it was? I was so excited when I heard his voice I thought I'd pass out.

"I can't believe you sent me your number," he said.

"Why not?"

"It just seems so, so... "

"So great?" I suggested.

"No. So forward."

"Forward?" Uh, oh. Was he one of those old-fashioned kind of guys? You know, cute, but a sexist jackass. Not that I'd care, mind you. Feminist movement be damned, if this guy could mambo (if you know what I mean) he could open all the doors for me he wanted.

"Yes. We've only been corresponding a short time." His response relieved me somewhat. He wasn't put off, he was shy.

"What are you talking about?" I argued calmly. "We've been exchanges messages for a month. How much longer were you planning to e-mail?"

"I don't know. I really love opening my mailbox and finding a note from you."

"Well, wouldn't you much prefer to open your front door and find me waiting for you?" He laughed at this for a long time. It wasn't that funny.

"I don't think my wife would like that very much."

"I'll come over when she's not around." This, too, was met with uncontrollable laughter.

"Oh come on, you wouldn't do that," he was chuckling.

"I would if you wanted me to," I said this very demurely. Of course I'd never go to his house. There were at least 25 perfectly good hotels in the downtown core with room service. No point getting lost in suburbia. I'd be too scared to ask a passerby for directions, for fear they might know the guy.

"I want to meet you. You're so funny," he said kindly.

"I want to meet you too. I like your e-mails, but you haven't made me laugh once. Are you always so serious?"

"No, not usually. You may have noticed that I am very shy."

Okay so that was his problem. I could vaguely remember him saying that it took him a while to feel comfortable around women.

"After a while you'll get used to talking to me, and I'll seem just like any other girl."

"I doubt you'll ever seem like that," he said, sounding bashful and uncertain.

"Well, call me every day at this time and you'll get to know me. Then you'll realize I can be a real pal." I tried to sound as reassuring as possible.

"Okay. I'll call every day."

I gave Rick my office number, because the free airtime on my cell doesn't kick in until after six. As promised, he called every day for six weeks solid. Finally having had enough of that, I asked him out to lunch. He agreed and we met the following week. He was stunningly gorgeous, and I thought there was no way in hell he could find me attractive. But he did. I knew this not because he said so, but because he called the next day, and the day after that, and the one after that. Then four weeks later when we met for lunch, we took the plunge. He booked a room at the Sheraton.

I met him in the parking lot. We were both so nervous we actually shook hands, which, considering what we were about to do, seemed really inappropriate and awkward. I'd brought along a briefcase with toiletries and clean underwear. It was a small guise so I'd appear to be attending a business meeting, rather than meeting my lover for sex *a la carte*. Rick didn't have any bags with him. All he carried was his wallet and a weak smile.

Rick hadn't checked in yet, so I had to stand in the lobby and wait. I wasn't sure whether to stand next to him, or off to the side, or over by the elevators. I decided on a position slightly to his left and about two feet behind him. The reservation girl kept trying to look at me, although she remained very courteous and professional. I guess my briefcase and cool business attire wasn't fooling her. It wasn't likely that Rick and I were the first people on the planet to rendezvous at the Sheraton.

I could hear Rick saying something about not wanting to use a credit card. I thought this was very smart. No sense in leaving a paper trail. I would have to remind him to discard the invoice the front desk clerk always presents you with during checkout. That should go directly in the garbage, but not in front of the hotel staff, because then they'd know for sure that we were lovers and that one of us, if not both, was married to someone else.

The reservation girl handed Rick the room key but when she said, "Have a pleasant stay," she looked right at me. Her face was a question mark of curiosity. Then it occurred to me that she might've thought I was a prostitute!

As soon as we were in the elevator, I said to Rick, "Oh my God, that girl thinks I'm a prostitute."

"Press twenty," he said and I obeyed.

"Rick, that girl thinks I'm a prostitute," I said, repeating myself.

"Well, of course she does, look at your little case," he gave my soft leather brief case a jab.

"Don't I look like a lawyer or something?"

"In that skirt? No," he gave me a lascivious grin. The look I was going for was sexy businesswoman. I didn't want to look like a librarian. Maybe I should have worn my glasses. But people in glasses don't have sex lives, at least not this kind. Do they?

As soon as we got to the room, I had to watch Rick fumble with the key. He was worse than Dakota. It was agonizing to watch a tall man fumble repeatedly with a simple hotel key. Add to this his stupid little chuckle each time the red light came on. For God's sake, couldn't he read a simple diagram? I wanted to show him how to do it, but I worried he might think I was a pro from experiences with other Ashley Madison men. On the contrary, this was my first time going to a hotel with a man who wasn't my husband. If this clumsy awkwardness was going to play out every time, I was better off with Dogbiscuit. If Dogbiscuit was with me, we would've been naked in the bed by now. Then again, I wouldn't have anything to look forward to, so I bit my tongue and remained quiet.

When Rick finally got the door open, I walked in, threw my leather case on the dresser and headed straight for the mini-bar. If ever there was a situation that demanded a stiff drink, this was it.

"What would you like?" I asked over my shoulder.

"What is there?"

"Rum, scotch, gin, whisky and a bottle of Chardonnay."

"I'll take a scotch over ice."

"Can you get some ice?"

"Where?"

Was he dumb or just nervous?

"There should be an ice machine down the hall." Oops, there I go, sounding like a pro.

"Yes, of course," he said. He left the room before I got up from the bar. There was a small fridge with four cans of pop and two bottles of water. I grabbed the 7-Up and poured it into a glass with some gin. I couldn't wait for the ice. I was nervous and dry mouthed and I needed the kind of courage you get from a bottle. There was a knock on the door, which sent my heart into my throat.

"Who is it?"

"It's Rick," came a voice with a distinct Irish lilt. Why had I never noticed his accent before?

I opened the door and couldn't keep the annoyance out of my voice.

"Why didn't you take the room key with you?"

"I meant to, but I forgot."

"Well you scared the shit out of me," I said, grabbing the bucket of ice. I made Rick a drink while he laughed at me.

"Why are you laughing?" I asked, really feeling the bite of anger rising in my chest.

"You," he doubled over again. He was sitting on the edge of the bed in hysterics. I went to the bed and pushed him over. That made him laugh harder. I went back to the mini-bar and drank, waiting for courage to arrive. When my glass was half empty, Rick sat up, straight-faced.

"Come here, sweetheart." He stretched his hands out toward me.

"I don't think so," I said, feeling embittered.

"You think I was laughing at you."

"You weren't?" I asked.

"Of course I wasn't. But you should have seen your..." he collapsed into yet another round of laughter. I finished my drink, and took a sip of the one I made for him. It burnt my throat so I'd made another gin and 7 for myself.

"Come here, buttercup. You know I'm absolutely crazy about you."

"I don't know anything of the sort. All I know is you've just wasted ten minutes of our precious afternoon together, laughing hysterically at nothing."

"Come over here, and I'll show you how sorry I am and how much I adore you."

I went to him, not because I was feeling forgiving, but because the two drinks were demanding I take a seat. When I reached the bed, Rick pulled me on top of him and that seemed like an even better idea. His mouth was soft and coaxing. His hands traveled expertly over my body, making me forget about his awkwardness with the room key, and the annoying way he laughs at everything. It was probably just nervous laughter anyway. It would disappear as soon as he was comfortable with me.

Rick's hands became more focused as his kisses deepened. His hands unzipped my skirt and slid the light, wool fabric over my hips. I kicked it to the floor. My blouse was next to go. All traces of Rick's awkwardness had vanished. I was lying in his arms wearing only my sensible Calvin Klein bra and panty set thinking, *More, more, more.*

I moved my hands to his waist and unzipped his pants. I slipped my hands inside and moved my fingers around. I couldn't feel anything, so I took my hand out and tried to undo his button. He brushed my hand away, deftly undid the button and in a fluid movement, removed his pants. There was no point in stopping at his boxers. I rolled over and positioned myself between his legs, so I could pull down his gray Jockeys over his hips and off his long legs. I slid my body off the edge of the bed as I did this. Then I got back on the bed to have a look at him. That's when I froze. The image of the little old lady from the hamburger commercials who used to demand from the startled counter attendant, "Where's the beef?" popped into my head. I bent closer. Now I've heard about small penises, but this was ridiculous. It looked like a cocktail wiener hiding beneath a bed of cilantro.

Rick raised himself up on his elbows, "What's the matter?" What's the matter? Was this guy for real? Why didn't he warn me?

"Uh, Rick," I said, searching for tact, which had walked out on me, "what's the matter with your dick?"

"Nothing, it'll grow. Come on, don't look at me like that."

He seemed so confident, I was momentarily torn. He obviously felt he could deliver the goods. Of course, with such a small delivery system it would probably take more than one trip. All of a sudden, I remembered a conversation I'd overheard in college between two girls I rarely hung out with. They were talking about a guy they'd both slept with once. I vaguely remember them having a chuckle over how small the guy was. But then they both asserted that, even though he wasn't well endowed, he was an incredibly good lover. Something about being quite adept at compensating orally for what he lacked genitally. Maybe it was a common trait amongst smaller guys. Rick had a pretty sly look on his face as if he was saying "I know something you don't know." If he was as good as he was making himself out to be, this might just turn out okay. So I thought *what the hell, as long as I'm already here*. In for a penny, in for a pound, or in this case, a quarter pound. I decided to ignore Rick's shortcomings (sorry) and gave him the benefit of the doubt. We resumed necking. His technique was certainly good. Well, it was better than Dogbiscuit's anyway. I wasn't really the best judge of male sexual ability. All I knew was that Dogbiscuit was the world's worst lover. Rick could be the second worst, for all I knew. But I was enjoying it, so I wasn't complaining. After about ten minutes, I felt Rick trying to nudge me down his torso by pushing on my shoulders.

"What's wrong?" I asked.

"Nothing," Rick replied. "I just want you to give a little T.L.C. to Ricky Jr." Oh God, it's true. Men do nickname them. Talk about too much time on your hands.

"Okay," I said. I didn't mind, as long as I got my fair share. "Why don't we do a little sixty-nine?"

"Sixty-nine? Ewww that's gross." I couldn't believe my ears.

"You aren't going to go down on me?"

"Ooh, yuck. I hate doing that. If you'd like, I can finger you a bit."

I was stunned. That was the best he could offer. A finger? I could do that myself for Christ's sake.

"You mean to tell me that you want me to give you oral sex, but you won't do the same for me. You expect that… that… cocktail wienie to do the trick?!" There, I said it. I was suddenly reminded of that old self-deprecating joke, "My girlfriend told me she wanted me to give her nine inches and make it hurt, so I fucked her three times and punched her in the nose." I was outraged. I got out of the bed and started gathering my clothes. "Listen, I don't know about you, but I don't believe in miracles."

"Sharon, Sharon, what are you doing?"

"Look Rick, I like you, but I already live with a train wreck. I don't need a circus freak for a lover."

"Sharon please, don't leave."

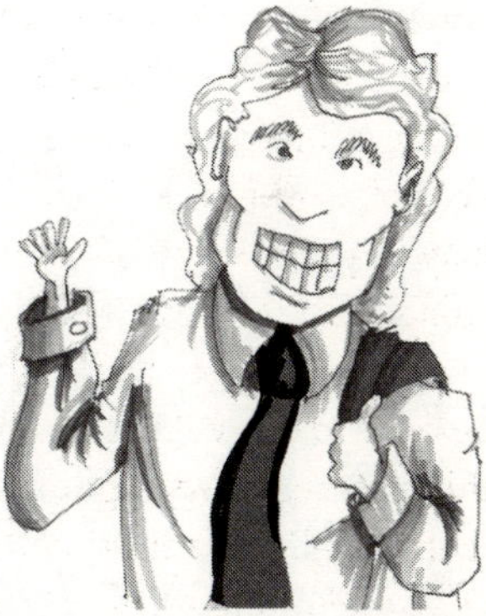

"Rick, I'm sorry," I said dressing quickly. "We've been in this room for over an hour. You're a wonderful kisser, but I want to play more adult games, and somehow I don't think you're up to it. Forgive the pun."

"Sharon, I can't believe you're upset because I'm small."

"Small I can handle. But you," I said, wagging an indignant finger, "you're microscopic. And to top it off, you're selfish. You were laughing at me, all the while you had your own joke hiding in your pants." Just as those words flew out of my mouth, that silly song by Sharon, Lois, and Bram popped into my head. Before I could stop myself, I blurted out, "I can't believe you'd let anyone see your skinamarinky dinky dick!"

With that, I closed the door and my mind to Carrick's warm embrace, and sweet kisses. As I walked down the corridor to the elevators, it occurred to me that I shouldn't have judged him so harshly. Maybe he was great in bed, just as his kisses had implied.

Once Gavin said to me "I just want you to know there are showers and there are growers." I didn't really get what he was talking about, and I was too embarrassed to ask. But once the elevator doors opened and I stepped in, I realized Carrick might have been a grower. For a second, I debated going back. Then the elevator doors closed and I was whisked to the lobby.

As I left the hotel, I kept my eyes averted from the reservation agents at the front desk. I did this to protect myself from their curios gazes as much as to shield my face from their view. One look at my unhappy face, and it would be apparent to even the most insensitive soul, that I didn't have a pleasant stay. And no, I wouldn't be coming again soon. I didn't come at all.

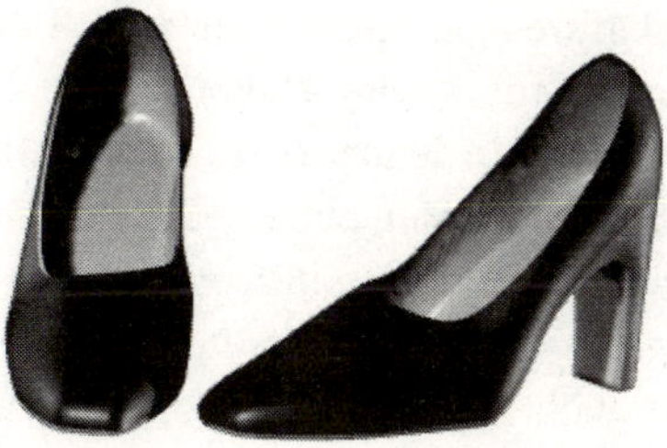

Chapter Four:
Elephant Man

I hadn't talked to Dakota in ages. I wanted to tell her everything about Carrick. I wouldn't mention Mike, because there was no need to dredge up that bit of rejection. I knew I should have gotten over it by then, but I hadn't. I was still mad. He shouldn't have said all those nice things if he wasn't sincere. As for Carrick, well he should come with a warning, "Objects in pants are smaller than you would imagine." There was, however, another guy I was dying to tell Dakota about.

I'd met him just when I thought I should take a break from MadAsh. I'd been on the system since March and now it was June, and I hadn't had any hot and heavy sex action yet. The mild petting and gentle caresses with Carrick were good, but I needed more. When Dakota and I first joined, I'd assumed that by summer, I'd be rolling around in 300-thread-count bedsheets with my Ashley Madison lover, assured of complete discretion. Surely I'd clocked enough hours on MadAsh. If there were justice in this world, I'd be deep in the groove of a relationship with my Internet hottie. I didn't expect instant gratification, but waiting this long felt like waiting for a fire to start from rubbing two damp sticks together.

Being the persistent trooper that I am, I didn't give up. I went online each and every day, and almost every night, in search of Mr. RightNow. It wasn't long before I was reeling in potential lover number three. His online name was Fit&Fabulous. I had only spoken to Fit a few times before agreeing to meet him. I didn't want to invest a lot of time in playing the getting-to-know-you game before meeting face to face. One thing I'd learned from my online episodes is that most men are far better lovers in cyberspace than in the space between me and the bedsheets. It no longer seemed wise to spend countless hours chatting on the phone or sending e-mails week after week. That's what I did with my first two hopefuls, and those potential relationships fizzled like defective Fourth of July firecrackers. I thought it was time for a new strategy. My new plan was: make contact, establish some common interests, meet, and make love. Fairly simple, and with any luck it would yield great results.

Fit sounded like a winner online, and that gave me a lot of hope. We were both really into our bodies. He built muscle and I burned fat. We were gym junkies to the extreme, although, my preferred method of burning fat involves platform heels and an afternoon at the mall. What really got my engine running was when Fit wrote, *Women tell me I look like a movie star.* Naturally a vision of a shirtless Mark Wahlberg popped into my head and stayed there the entire time I was instant messaging Fit. I had to cross my legs and squeeze after I read the following:

Fit&Fabulous: *Let's meet.*

I immediately sent back: SharonSharalike: *Okay.*

I was thinking third time has to be a winner. I agreed to meet Fit the next day for coffee at Starbucks. We settled on a 10:30 rendezvous, since I had to be at work by noon. Fit wanted me to meet him downtown. I was going to say yes, but then I remembered the downtown core was a maze of King Kong skyscrapers and people who always seem too busy to point you in the right direction. When I am downtown, I become really confused because there are no shop windows from which to take bearings. I mean, really, there should be a Gap store, an Old Navy, a Club Monaco, a Nordstrom, and a

Victoria's Secret. Without retail stores, I'm about as successful at navigating the downtown as a hillbilly from Little Rock, Arkansas in Times Square. I could just see myself sitting in one Starbucks waiting for Fit, while he sat in another on the next block, wondering what the hell had happened to me. I know for a fact this has happened to other Ashley Madison hopefuls.

One night, shortly after I received my Primus disc in the mail and had the Internet installed on my Dell laptop, I logged into MadAsh. In minutes, I was engaged in four really good instant messaging conversations. One guy, DoYou, told me he'd been stood up twice, by two different women. His first meeting was to take place at a Tim Horton's near Yonge and Eglinton. Now, I knew there were two Tim Horton's close to that intersection so I wrote, *Which one?* He said there was only one.

I sent the following message: *Ha Ha Ha.*

Then he asked me what was so funny. The rest of our conversation went like this:

SharonSharalike: *Loser, you weren't stood up. You went to the wrong place.*

DoYou: *What do you mean?*

SharonSharalike: *At that intersection there is a Tim's on Yonge and one on Eglinton. Which one did you go to?*

DoYou: *It doesn't matter now.*

SharonSharalike: *Tell me, anyway.*

DoYou: *Eglinton.*

SharonSharalike: *Ha Ha Ha.*

DoYou: *What's so funny now?*

SharonSharalike: *She was probably waiting for you at the Yonge location. Ha Ha.*

DoYou: *I doubt it. I was pretty clear about where I wanted to meet.*

SharonSharalike: *Maybe in your head, but obviously she thought something different.*

DoYou: *I dropped her, so I don't care where she was.*

SharonSharalike: *Well, what you should've done was change your name from DoYou, to Do-Fus.*

After that, he wouldn't talk to me. I focused on my other three conversations without an ounce of remorse. Better luck next time, DoYou.

For my meeting with Fit, I wanted to be precise about location, so I selected the Starbucks in Chapters on Bloor Street. I told him to find me in the magazine racks.

So, there I was, on Tuesday morning, having a clothing fit in my walk-in closet. I stared at all my clothes, dumbfounded. So much stuff, and yet I still felt I had nothing to wear. There were racks and racks of shirts and blouses. Below the tops were skirts hung according to length, and beside those were my dresses, grouped according to level of formality. All my high-end stuff is at the back of the closet, so when you walk in the first thing you see is Chanel, Dolce & Gabana, Donna Karan, Ralph Lauren, and Calvin Klein. So far, I only have one item by each designer, but there's plenty of room for more. I just have to figure out a way to get Dogbiscuit to loosen his hold on the purse strings.

My clothing dilemma arose because I wanted to look sexy for my meeting with Fit, but I also had to look business casual for work after my date. Plus, I had to get past Margaret on my way out the door. Anything too racy would cause her to smirk, or worse, pass some kind of sarcastic remark that would send me running back to my closet like a thirteen-year-old preparing for her first dance. After careful deliberation, I settled on a black and white hound's tooth skirt. It had become a mini when I failed to heed the DRY CLEAN ONLY label. Who knew water could have such a dramatic affect on a garment. Anyway, I much prefer my skirt in this new size. I have to watch my weight though, because it fits me like a glove. I paired the skirt with a black sweater set. I thought I looked very smart and sexy too. A long silver necklace provided the ooh-la-la the outfit needed.

By the time I was dressed, it was already 9:45. That meant my hair had to go up in a ponytail instead of the French twist the outfit called for. By the time I'd applied make-up, it was 10:05, which meant I was going to be late. I got to Chapters at 10:45. Ten minutes late is no biggie, even fifteen minutes is forgivable. Dogbiscuit is put out if he has to wait two minutes, but I think most men are fairly reasonable about time. At least that's what I told myself as I headed up the escalator toward the magazine racks.

When I got there, the area was actually empty. I picked up a *Honey* and leafed through it. When I looked up there were some other people around, but no one who looked like Marky Mark. I returned the

Honey and grabbed a *Cosmopolitan*. I held it in my hand and read the cover first. There's always so much good sex advice. I couldn't decide if I should read about the sex games or how to interpret his body language. Since there weren't too many people around, and since my number three might actually turn out to be the one, I opted for the sex games. My fingers had just found the right page when a voice behind me made me turn around sharply.

"Excuse me?" he said. He was a really tall version of Bryan Adams.

"Yes," I said wishing, and hoping he was Fit, even though he was too tall and two thin to match the description.

"I hope this doesn't offend you, but you're really gorgeous. I just came over to tell you that." He smiled and I smiled back. I wondered if Mike knew what a hot commodity he'd passed up when he decided not to call me again.

"Thank you," I said, feeling sincerely flattered.

"You're welcome, the pleasure was all mine. I'm Andrew," he held out his hand. I shook it.

"Nice meeting you, Andrew. I'm Sharon."

"Do you come here often, Sharon?"

"Err, no," I said. Maybe it was time to consider an alternate route to work. I could breeze by Chapters every morning to see who I might attract. Maybe there was a George Clooney look-alike out there somewhere. If there was, I wanted first dibs on him.

"Well, perhaps I'll meet you here again."

"Sure," I said scrunching my perfectly arched brows together. Was he trying to tell me something? Was he saying to meet him here again tomorrow? Or was he just trying to transform a compliment into a conversation?

"Take care," he said.

"Thank you, I will," I said. I was thinking he could probably take care of me in all the right ways, know what I mean? You should've seen his swagger as he walked off.

I looked around the magazine area wondering if Fit had come and gone. Then a man in a Boston blue shirt approached me.

"Sharon?"

"Yes. Are you Fit?"

"I am." Okay, what happened to Mark Wahlberg? Fit said he was built, which he was. The shirtsleeves were positively rippling with sinewy muscles. His tie, which didn't match the shirt unless you were color blind, sat in the valley between two perfectly formed pectoral muscles. The body, at least the upper part was a perfect ten. But when I looked into his face, he didn't even bear a distant resemblance to the star of the revisited *Planet of the Apes.* I even tried to squint and use my imagination.

"What's your real name?" I should have asked yesterday when we were chatting. Note to self: Don't rush into meetings without some basic knowledge of the person you're scheduled to meet.

"Richard," he said, and held his hand out. I shook it.

"It's great to meet you Richard, or should I say Dick?"

"No, don't call me that. Call me Richard."

"Okay," I said, trying to ignore the testy note in his voice. Lots of people shorten Richard to Dick. The fact that he didn't like it might mean something. I just wasn't sure what. In my current state of sex deprivation, calling every man I met Dick sounded like a great idea.

"Do you want to head over to Starbucks for a coffee?" he asked, looking down at me. At least he was about Mark Wahlberg's height, I think.

"Sure, but I don't drink coffee during the summer. I'd prefer a frappaccino."

"Okay, I'll have one too. Are they any good?" Are they good? What planet did this guy sail in from?

"Yes. You've never had one?"

"Nope," he said without an ounce of shame or a hint of regret.

"Well, Richard, you're in for a real treat." If he didn't like his frappaccino, I'd drop him like a maxed out credit card.

We walked into Starbucks and Richard gestured that I should take a seat. I sat down at a small, clean-looking table and hung my purse strap over the chair back. I looked around the coffee shop. At the table behind us a girl was studying something that looked related to math. By the fireplace, there were people in business apparel lounging on the sofas. Richard came over with the drinks and two wrapped straws. I thanked him, then got up and grabbed a couple of napkins. It was my mother's instinct to always prepare for a spill, although I have no idea where those instincts were the night I spilled nail polish on Dogbiscuit's Persian rug.

I handed a napkin to Richard and sat down. Now that I was sitting across from him, I could have a really good look. Maybe too good a look. I don't know who told Richard he looked like a movie star, but whoever said it must have been referring to John Hurt when he played John Merrick, in *The Elephant Man*. Richard stripped the wrap from his straw and stuck it in his plastic cup. He pulled deeply on his straw and when the frappaccino entered his mouth his face lit up.

"Do you like it?" I asked.

"It's great. I wonder how many calories it's got," he looked at the cup as if he was calculating the kilojoules.

"I think it's fairly low fat, so no worries."

"Well, one of these, once in a while, won't hurt," he said, taking another long sip. God, he was worse than me with the calorie counting.

"Are you very careful about what you eat?" I asked, already knowing the answer.

"Yes, I basically only eat raw." Oh brother, I can't handle anyone who is more food phobic than me.

"Really, so basically you eat lettuce and carrot sticks?" He laughed before taking another sip. Maybe I could convert him to a high calorie, saturated fat friendly, reduced fiber, processed rich diet.

"This is really good." His drink was more than half gone. I guess if you only drink cabbage juice and water, a frappaccino would taste like a row of pink diamonds. Astounding.

Richard started to tell me about his special diet. He eats the same five meals every day. If you think that sounds dull, you should hear him explain it. While he spoke, I kept my eyes riveted to his face, and that's probably why I noticed there was something disproportionate about Richard. I looked at him, while he went on and on about the virtues of raw cauliflower, thinking his neck was awfully big. It was about the size of the fattest part of my thigh. I started to wonder if his fabulously developed body was maybe a little too developed, if you know what I mean.

"Richard, do you get your shirts custom made?"

"Some are. Not all of them."

"Is that one?" I said pointing with my drink.

"Yes," he said patting his tie. "Have you ever considered getting a juicer?" Oh God, was he back on that again?

"Yes," I said even though the thought had never once crossed my mind. That set Richard off on the topic of what I should look for in a good juice machine. To my way of thinking, a good juice machine is any guy who looks like Mark Wahlberg. His body gets me fired up every time.

Now Richard's body was really good too, but something wasn't in balance. I looked over his chest and even though the tie was making me dizzy, his upper body was faultless. I took a long sip of my drink. The icy coolness was a welcome relief to my hot mouth.

"Sharon?" I looked up at Richard. His face was a giant question mark. Oops! I hoped I hadn't said anything aloud.

"Yes?"

"Well?"

"Well, what?"

"I asked if you wanted me to help you out with a new diet regime."

"Can I steam my vegetables?"

"Sure, it's important to eat some things raw, but you don't have to eat everything that way."

"Good, because raw broccoli gets stuck in my teeth. Especially the front ones." That made Richard laugh. When he lifted his head slightly, he totally obliterated my view of the sun. It was a total eclipse. In that moment of darkness, the light came on in my head and I realized that what was wrong with Richard had nothing to do with his truly well-defined body, and everything to do with his enormous head.

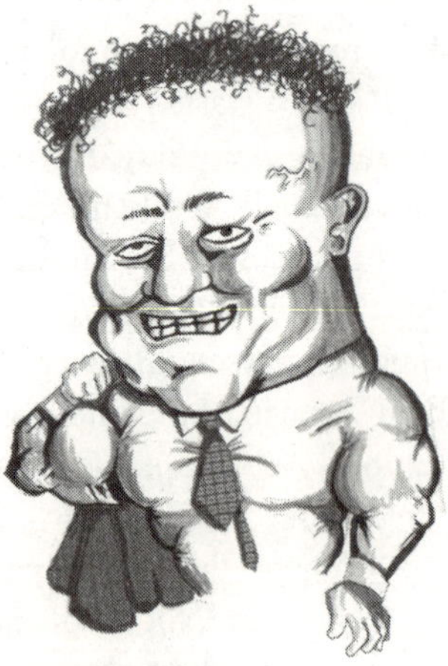

I'd never seen a head so big. It was, as my son would say, "gi-normous". In fact, if Richard's neck hadn't been so big, his head would've snapped it like a twig and rolled off his shoulders. I was tempted to ring Dogbiscuit on my mobile phone, to come round and have a look at this oddity. Dogbiscuit, believing he is beyond reproach, loves to look at human abnormalities. He would definitely get a kick out of Richard's head, and he'd probably notice it right away. It took me a full twenty-three minutes to finally figure out what was off about Richard. I couldn't take my eyes off his face. What could have done this to him?

Before I could stop myself, I asked him,"Richard, how many pounds did you weigh at birth?"

"What?'

"Err, nothing," I might as well let it go. I doubt he was anything like that baby I read about in the *National Enquirer.*

"I'm sorry I missed what you said. Did you want to know where I was born?"

"Yes," I said.

"I was born in Grand Rapids," blah, blah, blah. He was boring even when he wasn't talking about food. I couldn't concentrate on anything he said because his head had taken over. I couldn't see around that thing.

"How do you get out of bed?" I asked.

"What?"

"I was just wondering how you raise yourself from prone position?" Wasn't that what ultimately killed the Elephant Man? He tried to lie down and his head snapped his neck. I think that's what happened in the movie. Now Michael Jackson owns the carcass. That's just too weird to even contemplate.

"I get out of bed like everyone else. Why? What do you do?"

"Well, some people," I put a slight emphasis on some, "lift themselves into a sitting position first then swing their legs over the edge. Other people," I gave him a meaningful look, "literally roll out of bed."

"I think I sit up." He looked puzzled.

"Oh," I said slightly disappointed. It would have been much more interesting to hear about how he struggled with his enormous head to lift himself out of bed.

"You must have strong stomach muscles," I told Richard.

His face colored slightly and then he said, "Would you like to see them?"

I smiled."Yes, but not just now." Frankly, I can't handle any more excitement for one day.

"I bet you have good stomach muscles too," he said. I almost choked on my frappaccino. After boring me for three-quarters-of-an-hour, he just now thought of pouring on the charm.

"I do," I said proudly. No one likes false modesty, so I might as well be honest.

"You and I should work out together. Would you be interested in coming to my gym some time?"

"Sure," I said. Honestly, I'm not into working out with other people. When I go to the gym with Dakota, all we do is talk and try out equipment we have no idea how to use. Typically we run for fifteen minutes, cycle for twenty, stretch for twenty, sit on the universal machines for thirty, shower and leave. That's our two-hour workout routine. Without Dakota, I workout twice as much in half the time. Even so, I don't think I'm up to Richard's standards.

"Great, what are you doing on Saturday?" he said, expecting an immediate yes from me. I hoped to be having sex on Saturday with someone I was attracted to. That would exclude both Dogbiscuit and Richard.

"I don't know, it's only Tuesday," I said, thinking I had only four days to make my wish come true. Could I find a guy that fast?

"Well, why don't I call you on Thursday to see if you're free?"

"How about if I call you?"

"That would be fine. We can have lunch after our workout."

"Okay," I said. I didn't like the way he said workout. Some guys think you should really sweat it up in the gym. I didn't want Richard pushing me beyond what I could endure. I'm not up for power step and boot camp experiences. I like the kind of exercise you do in a sitting position, like trying on shoes, or cycling. Or those wonderful exercises that tone, strengthen, and shape your body while you're lying down. I know this sounds like I'm talking about Pilates, but no. Pilates would be ideal, but every two seconds you have to throw your legs in the air, and you're not allowed to relax them to the ground. You have to control your movements, which puts unbearable strain on your stomach muscles, and thighs. Personally, I'm into less painful ways to shape my hips, butt, and thighs.

Yoga once seemed like the working girl's answer to exercise. It should be ideal, because the simple form of this exercise is actually the cool down portion of more vigorous exercise classes, like kick boxing. The problem with yoga is there's too much work on balance and not enough focus on lying down and listening to the harmony of your beating heart.

The best exercise from a prone position has to be sex. When it's done correctly, you not only burn calories, you can really reduce the size of your thighs too. Dakota tells me that some of the positions she's tried by mimicking her favorite porn videos, can induce a thigh burn and an orgasm. That beats both Pilates and yoga.

Anyway, even if I were to survive a workout with Richard, I didn't think I could get through an entire meal with this guy. That was asking an awful lot. I mean just getting together for coffee was tough enough. First off, he was boring. Secondly, his head was too big.

"I know quite a few good restaurants that are open for lunch," he said, trying to coax a commitment from me. That's nice. I wanted to tell him I too knew a few good restaurants. I could also think of about one hundred other people I'd prefer to dine with, including the vagrant I'd passed on my way into Chapters that morning.

"I should get going now, but I'll call you." I started to get up to leave.

"You'll need my number."

"Oh yeah," I said smiling brightly. "I can't leave without that."

"Yeah, good thing for Ashley, because you can always get in touch with me there."

"Right," I said, waiting as he searched his pockets for a pen. He wrote his number down on the Starbucks' napkin, folded it twice, and handed it to me. I slipped it into my purse.

"Thanks for the frappaccino and the advice about the juice." I couldn't remember anything else Richard had talked about, because my attention had been hijacked by the size of his head.

"No problem, Sharon" he said smiling. His teeth weren't bad, but his smile made his head seem even wider.

When I walked out of Chapters, the umpire in my head called out, "Strike three!"

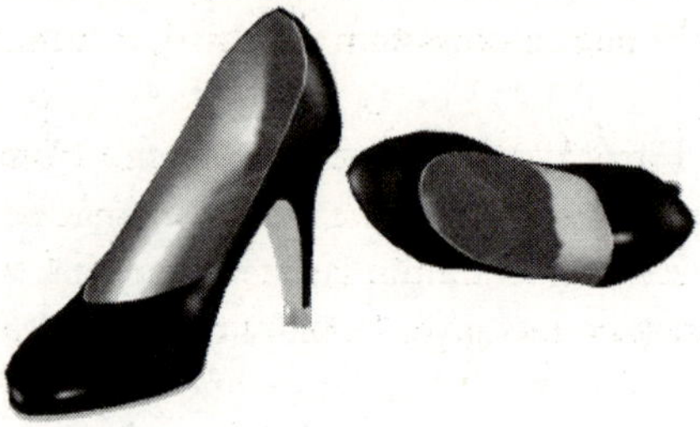

Chapter Five:
Panty Man

I needed sexual healing that day. Instantly. I was on edge. I couldn't relax and the slightest things made me go postal. I really needed to get my groove on with a guy who was at least halfway handsome. Any day, Dogbiscuit was going to roll over in bed and put his bony hand on my hip. When he did, how would I refuse him? I hadn't had sex in... four, five... seven months! Oh my God, how could I go on? I was weak in the knees. My hands shook, rattled, and rolled each time I reached for my glass of Perrier. Pretty soon, people were going to start wondering why I was impersonating Katherine Hepburn. When I tried to speak, most of my words came out as gibberish. Ozzy Osbourne was more coherent.

If that wasn't bad enough, everything reminded me of sex. Not just smokestacks and dental instruments, even simple things like ice-cream cones and hot dogs. And the damn TV guide was filled with subliminal images; have you ever noticed how many futon and home sauna ads they run? If I didn't have sex soon, I'd degenerate like

Charlie in *Flowers for Algernon.* I had to save myself. I had to get serious online. No more fooling around making idle chit-chat with men I was never going to meet. I had to find a sex partner. It was a matter of life and health.

The trouble was, apart from Carrick and Mike, I hadn't been able to connect with anyone I was attracted to. If Elephant Man had a better head, say four sizes smaller, maybe we could have worked around the fact that his face was the kind that encourages you to keep your eyes closed. As it was, I had to cross him and his big, beautiful biceps off my list.

Speaking of Carrick, I'd received a message from him the night before. I was tempted to give him the second chance he requested, but then I thought better of it. I didn't send a reply. I was hoping my silence would carry the message. I wasn't desperate enough to revisit Dinky.

I had been the night before, but then I was inundated with instant messages. I could not keep up. Just for the record, I seemed to be growing in popularity. Some nights, everyone wanted a piece of me. I mean this literally. I'd had a few online spats lately. It wasn't my fault. My sexual deprivation was turning me into an extraordinary bitch. I was so abrasive, I expected to grow satanic horns. In fact, on one Monday, I snapped at Ralph so severely, he jumped. I had to make it up to him, so during my lunch break, I asked him about his weekend.

"Oh," Ralph said, moving cranberry bread around in his mouth so he could speak, "it was really, really good." We were seated side by side around the rectangular lunch table.

"Really?" I asked. How could Ralph have had a weekend so fantastic he had to use two "reallys" to describe it?

"Yup," he said taking another bite of his neatly sliced bread. I wondered if Ralph baked his snacks himself.

"Remember that girl I told you about a couple of weeks ago?" No, I didn't.

"Yeah, the cute one you sort of liked," I said, expertly covering for my complete and total lack of recall. It was a pretty safe bet that the girl was cute. It wasn't likely Ralph would be telling me about some skank. No one talks about ugly women anyway; not even ugly men. That's the problem with being unattractive—it renders you invisible, but not the good kind of invisible that allows you to shoplift and spy undetected in the dressing rooms of the opposite sex.

"Well, guess what?" Ralph asked, swallowing the last bit of cranberry bread.

"What?"

"She came over."

"Over where?"

"Over to my place," Ralph said. He made an attempt to roll his eyes. His irises got stuck at the top so he looked like he was staring at the ceiling. Maybe he was, I looked up too, then back at him.

"What did you two do?"

"I made dinner, and then we got it on," Ralph said, trying to sound like Barry White. Yeah sure, Ralph having hot monkey sex. I'd believe that when I saw it. Not that I'd ever want to see it. Just thinking about him with an erection was enough to make me want to end the conversation. The last thing I wanted to hear about was Ralph's escapade as Casanova. It wasn't right that he got to have sex and I didn't. Furthermore, I didn't want to hear Ralph talking about what he ate for dinner while I was suffering through hunger pangs on my current get-lean-so-you-will-look-gorgeous-naked diet. Unfortunately, curiosity propelled me forward.

"No you didn't," I said to Ralph, skepticism written on my face. I only had four grapes left and I was still hungry. My stomach growled and I looked up at Ralph apologetically. There were a few crumbs left from his cranberry bread. I was tempted to scrape them into my palm and throw them in my mouth. Yes, I was that hungry. Two rice cakes, a bottle of water, and fourteen grapes is more than a snack, but less than a lunch. A lot less.

"Oh, yes we did," Ralph nodded his head.

"Wow, what did you feed her?" I actually meant that as a joke, but Ralph took me seriously.

"Oh, I ordered in, Japanese," he said smiling. He looked like he'd just convinced another celebrity to run for political office, which always seems like a good idea until the celebrity wins.

"Right," I said thinking about raw fish on a plate. Is that a highly sexual image, or is it just me? "I think I read somewhere that raw fish is an aphrodisiac." Or is it fish eggs?

"Bingo," Ralph snapped his fingers and pointed at me.

"But it's not all raw fish, there's a certain type right?"

"Duh, of course. I wasn't going to serve her mackerel."

"Yes, I know, but tuna fish isn't going to do it for you either." Ralph started laughing. When he stopped, it didn't seem like he was going to say anything further, so I prompted him.

"What did you serve?"

"Oh, I just ordered one of those sushi platters."

"Right, how did you know what to order?"

"Why the third degree? You planning a little romantic night with hubby?" Ralph gave me a wink and a nudge. If only he knew.

"Listen Ralph," I said leaning towards him, "it would take a lot more than a Bento box of raw fish to get my husband pumped up."

Ralph stared at me blankly for a moment then he said, "That's too bad. You know there's always Viagra."

"It's very expensive," I said. I know that because one day on my way in to work I listened to the morning health show on the radio and the topic was Viagra. The guest medical expert had claimed there was only one downside to the drug and that was cost. Other than that, he argued that Viagra was not only safe and effective, it was also as beneficial as aspirin.

"Is it?" Ralph asked, wide-eyed. I nodded. "Figures, anything that works costs money."

"How do you know it works?"

"It's gotta work. Just about every man over fifty-five is on it. Didn't you hear about Phil in accounting?"

"No," I said positively beaming. I hadn't heard a shred of gossip in months. Ever since I joined Ashley Madison, my head had been glued to my computer screen.

"Phil had some Viagra prescribed by his doctor, and it worked so well he traded his fifty-year-old wife in for two twenty-five-year-olds." Ralph started to laugh uncontrollably.

"That's such a tired old joke, it isn't even funny anymore."

"Sure it is," he said, between his hee-haws.

"No it isn't."

"Well, it's a true story. Not the trading part, but Phil is divorcing his wife."

"What about the Viagra?"

"That's true too."

"Well, I once heard," I leaned forward, proud that I'd remembered a long-forgotten bit of useless gossip, "that some guy took it and stayed hard for two hours."

"Where did you hear that?" Ralph was dubious.

"I don't remember. Maybe I saw it on TV." Actually, come to think of it, the two hours might be the punch line to a joke. I used to have a good memory, then I had children and deterioration set in. At times like this, I envy those who opt for pets instead of kids.

"I doubt anything is that potent." Ralph was clearly warming to the subject.

"Well, you probably don't need anything like that," I said, making an obvious attempt at flattery.

"No, I don't. And I certainly wouldn't want any, if it was going to cost me my marriage."

"Ralph, you're not married."

"I mean, if I were," he let out an exasperated sigh.

"Listen Ralph," I said moving closer, as if I was going to whisper something in his ear. "Viagra can't destroy a marriage. If Phil and his wife are breaking up, I'm sure they have a lot of irreconcilable differences. Sex is only part of their problem."

"I wouldn't be too sure about that," Ralph said. He started to pick at his own crumbs. My stomach grumbled again. I filled it with bottled water. I should've packed a Slim Fast shake. Then I could have pretended my rice cakes were two all-beef patties.

"Ralph, you've never been married. You have no idea what it feels like to be chained to another person."

"Marriage is a partnership between two people."

"In theory, yes, but you know what? I didn't get a partner, I got a paperweight."

Ralph started laughing.

"Is your husband a big-assed couch potato?"

"No, he's just a big ass." That brought more laughter. "Actually Ralph, it's no laughing matter. There are days when I wonder what the hell I did to deserve such punishment."

"You think of your marriage as punishment?"

"A life sentence."

"You shouldn't feel that way."

"Well, that's how I do feel."

"But only when you're mad or upset with your husband, right?"

"No, always."

Ralph couldn't bear to look at me any more, so he looked down at the table.

"Let me give you some sage advice, Ralph; don't get married."

"Sharon, everyone gets married sometime. That's the point of dating."

"Ralph, the point of dating is to find someone you get along with reasonably well, so you can get your groove on." This sent Ralph into another fit of hysterical laughter.

"So you think dating is all about sex?"

"Pretty much. I figure, if women didn't need to have sex, they wouldn't bother with men."

"That's crazy talk."

"Ralph, it's the truth."

"Well, I can't handle your version of the truth. I think people date for sex, but," he held up a finger, "companionship is a greater drive. That's why people marry."

"Only fools marry. Smart people know that marriage is like roller blading, doing a handstand, or eating with chopsticks; it looks easy until you try it."

"I think you can have a successful marriage if you find the right person."

That made me pause for a moment.

"It's possible," I conceded. "But how on earth do you find the right person?"

"You found yourself a husband so you must know something about it."

"Yeah, I now know what not to do." We both laughed.

"It's hard to find somebody. I know that. I didn't date anyone for about two years. Then I met Veronica, and I felt like I'd died and gone to heaven."

"That's the girl you invited to your place on the weekend?"

"Yes, I think I made a good impression. She seemed to have a good time."

"She could've been faking."

"Sharon!"

"Just a thought," I said, not meaning to be hurtful. After all, she could have been. "Here's some more advice Ralph."

"I didn't ask for any."

"Too bad, it's free, so you have to listen."

"Okay," he grumbled. I could almost hear the mental hum he started to block out my words.

"Ralph, listen to me, what do bigamy and monogamy have in common?"

"What?"

"They both occur when you have one spouse too many!"

You should have seen Ralph's face. He just stared at me. "I can't believe you're so pessimistic."

"Actually, I consider myself a realist."

"Okay, well the reality is that only half of all marriages end in divorce."

"And the other half grin and bear it." I put on my biggest shit-eating grin for emphasis.

"I liked you better when you scowled all day."

"No, you didn't," I said with the insane joker's smile on my face.

"Yeah, I did."

"Just trying to make you wiser, buddy," I said, sliding my lips back together. My jaws were sore. I had no idea smiling could be so painful. No wonder Dogbiscuit abstains.

"I'm sorry your marriage is so rotten it's left you jaded and irrational."

"Actually, I was jaded and irrational before I met my husband. My marriage only confirmed my bleak and dismal outlook on love and romance. Anyway, my marriage isn't bad, Ralph. It's lonely."

"Oh," he said. His face mirrored my feelings.

"No worries, Ralph. I'm a big girl, I can take care of myself. Maybe I'll find a Veronica of my very own."

"Let's hope you find yourself a Victor."

"Right," I said, getting up. Lunch was over and I was starving.

I had begun my Ashley Madison adventure with Dakota and I still hadn't talked to her in weeks. Every time I thought I had a few moments to give her a call, something came up. I was going to ring her after my date with Elephant Man. Dogbiscuit was scheduled to be away from home on Saturday for a golf game with his college buddies, but rained all day and the game was canceled. Dogbiscuit moped around the house the entire morning and then started shadow golfing. That really got on my nerves, so at around two o'clock, I packed up the kids and took them to the mall.

On Sunday we all went to church. By we, I mean me, the kids and my mom. Dogbiscuit's idea of regular church attendance means he never misses Christmas or Easter. The sermon was all about faith, including being faithful. Was God trying to tell me something? Was he telling me to hang on while He found the right Ashley Madison guy for me? I sure hoped so. Our house was jammed with people that Sunday afternoon. My mother likes to have a tea social once a month at my house, because it's larger than hers, and it bugs the shit out of Dogbiscuit. Even though I wasn't responsible for any of the entertaining, I had to be visible. Dogbiscuit insisted I keep my eyes on the valuables.

"There are thieves in every walk of life. Why should Christians be any different?"

"Because they're devout Christians," I hissed at him.

"Do you know where the highest percentage of Christians is clustered?"

"Where?"

"San Quentin."

"You're nuts," I said, walking away from him.

"Cover the front rooms. I'll watch the back."

I ignored him and I slipped into the living room to exchange a few pleasantries with the four ladies gathered on the chintz sofas. Why must they curl their hair so tightly? They looked like a herd of sheep in pastel dresses.

The first chance I got, I tiptoed upstairs. There were people admiring my daughter's bedroom as if this was an open house. There was absolutely no opportunity for me to call Dakota. I'd have to wait yet another week before I had a chance to tell her everything.

I was reluctant to call Dakota from work, because I wasn't using the office phone for personal calls anymore. When Ralph and I bonded over lunch the week before, I'd made a vow not only to be nicer to him, but also to obey some of the office rules. I'd been on time for work ever since, and with the exception of my hotel rendezvous with Dinky, I hadn't missed a single day at the office. During breaks, I was only taking the time allotted to me. No more forty-five-minute lunches followed by fifteen minutes in the washroom reapplying makeup. I only had thirty minutes each day and I was sticking to that.

As such a model citizen, I even reduced my swearing to lighthearted expletives when the photocopier jammed or when I had to wait more than fifteen seconds for the elevator. A pretty big improvement. The old me used to push on the down button frantically as though that would ensure the elevator's swift arrival. It never worked, but all the same, I'd huff and puff and press with enough force to turn that button from an "outie" to an "innie". I am so much calmer now. I've even started to solve problems on my own, rather than joining the office pool of complaints.

And rather than complain, I brought a sweater to work so I no longer have to curse at the thermostat. It's so fucking cold in that office. I think the company is trying to pick up a few extra bucks storing meat. Who sets that thing? They probably can't see how low it is because their breath fogs up their view of the needle. If it doesn't warm up around my desk by the end of next week, I'm putting brandy in the water cooler.

What I was most proud of, however, was the reduction in the amount of time I spent on the phone engaged in personal calls. That sincere effort to limit my phone use should make me a shoe-in to win employee of the month. Take that, receptionist who always has the homemade tollhouse cookies! I spent a lot of time on the Ashley Madison website, so I didn't actually have any time to call girlfriends.

The downside was that I couldn't talk to Dakota. I missed her and I was dying to know what she'd been up to. I decided to call Dakota during my lunch break. I figured, why not? It wasn't like I was wasting time eating food, unless you call half a Melba toast and two ounces of drained tuna, food. Dakota picked up on the first ring, which was good because I didn't feel like making small-talk with Kal.

"Hey, Dee how are you?"

"What's up, girlfriend?"

"Listen, I have so much to tell you," I said, lowering my voice. In an office you can never tell who might be eavesdropping.

"Oh yeah? Have you done it?"

"Yes," I said, even though I wasn't sure what it was.

"Me too!" Dakota squealed with delight, and I thought she might be jumping up and down on her blond maple floors. "When, where, who, and how many positions?"

"Err, do you want to go first?" I was thinking "it" was a blind date, but from what Dakota had just said, "it" sounded like a home run.

"Yeah, okay. I met him on the Internet."

"Ashley Madison?"

"Yes, of course. I still have Kal, you know." The way she said Kal, made him sound like a favorite pair of old jeans you don't wear anymore, but don't have the heart to throw away. Let's not forget Kal has the kind of body that should be placed securely between a woman's thighs. Ride 'em cowboy.

"Yes, I know you still have Kal," I said.

"It's been going really well."

"What? Are you in a relationship?"

"Well, not as such. I meet him every Wednesday morning."

"Every Wednesday?" I was incredulous.

"Pretty much," she said, and I could actually hear the smile on her face.

"When did all this start?"

"Um... he was the fourth guy I met."

Hmm… the fourth guy she met. That meant there was still hope for me. Yeah!

"So how long has it been going on?"

"About six weeks."

"Oh my God. Six weeks? And you haven't said a word to me? That's so not right."

"Well, he's really hot, but..."

"But he's married?" That sent us both into hysterical laughter. I almost peed because I had to be really quiet, and Dakota's laugh always makes me laugh more.

"No, no," Dakota said, when she recovered. "He *is* married, but that's not the but."

"Is he butt ugly?"

"No, remember Simon from Abnormal Psych?" As if I would ever forget Simon. Dakota and I sat behind him for an entire year, lusting after him. Eventually, Dakota moved on and found other men to occupy her time, but I never stopped fantasizing about Simon. Never.

"Does he have black hair, green eyes, and dark skin?" I asked, not really wanting my suspicion confirmed.

"Yes."

"Dakota, please don't tell me your guy looks like Simon."

"He does look like Simon." Okay that was it. That was the last straw. Why did Dakota always have to one-up me?

"I have to go now," I told her, getting ready to return the receiver to the cradle.

"No you don't. Shut-up and listen. He looks like Simon, but he isn't anything like him." We never actually found out what Simon was like, but between us, we created this marvelous profile of his sexy single life.

"What's your guy like, and what's his name?" I'd resigned myself to listen to her after all.

"Kevin. How sexy is that?"

"What's this thing you have for guys whose names start with K?"

"I know. Weird, huh?"

"I'll say," I couldn't be involved with two men with the same first initial. Imagine if I had to keep things straight between Dilbert and Dogbiscuit. It wouldn't work out.

"Anyway, Kevin is great!" Was that supposed to make me feel better?

"What's so great about him?" I asked. I was looking through my inbox for some work to complete while Dakota talked. I wasn't going to listen. I'd become a master at interjecting a "hmm", and an "uh huh", to make her believe I was all ears while I actually focused on something else. I found some corrections that had to be made to a document.

I got my copy pencil and had begun circling just as I heard Dakota say, "There's this weird thing about him."

"Oh?" I said. My pencil froze. "What might that be?"

"You can't tell a soul," she said whispering.

"I won't tell anyone," I whispered back.

"Okay, after the first time we did it, he asked me if I'd be okay with role-playing."

"And you said…?"

"I said, sure. So he said he wanted to try being the woman and he wanted me to pretend to be the man."

"Okay, that's weird."

"No, that's not the weird part."

"Really?" I would've been checking out of the hotel and waking a judge for a restraining order at that point. Who wants to be involved with a guy who wants to be a woman? That's not an actual life experience, it's the Jerry Springer show.

"He wanted us to wear each other's clothes."

"Did you?"

"Well, he couldn't get into my skirt, but he looked all right in my tank top."

"How did you look in his clothes?"

"I think normal, because he wore jeans and a golf shirt."

"Oh, how boring," I said.

"Yeah, so I had to be the man."

"How droll."

"No, it was so fun. You should try it."

"I can't imagine ever wanting to be a man. Did he put on your lipstick?"

"No, he's not into makeup or anything. It's just the clothes he likes."

"Okay, so how did the date end?" I said, doing my impression of Chuck Woolery from Love Connection.

"Don't freak out or anything, but we had so much fun. I got to boss him around and he pretended to be intimidated by my masculinity. We've been playing the same game week after week."

"The same game? Aren't you bored?" When I think of playing the same game over and over, a vision of Candyland pops into my head. I've played that game so much I actually hate candy now, especially candy canes and sugarplums, whatever the hell they are.

"No, but..."

"But what?" I asked.

"The but is, we don't wear each other's clothes anymore."

"Why not? Isn't that part of the whole tactile eroticism?"

He said he was afraid my perfume might rub off on his clothes or my hair might catch on his shirt and his wife might find it.

"I see."

"Anyway, we still role-play, but all he wants to do is wear my underwear."

"Does that include your bras?"

"No."

"How about your thongs?"

"Yes," Dakota sounded like she was confessing a sin to her parish priest.

"That is just disgusting," I said, affecting a self-righteous tone.

"Do you see why I haven't called you?"

"Isn't he stretching your underwear out?"

"You know what? He actually snapped the elastic on one. And he continued to pretend that he was a girl even though one side was hanging off his hairy ass." That made us both squeal with laughter. I couldn't stop myself. I didn't care who heard.

"After that, you had sex with him?" I said wiping the tears from my eyes.

"Yes, he's really cute."

"Does he play this game with his wife?"

"No, of course not. That's what brought him online. He can't even tell her about his fantasy."

"Well, it is kind of weird. Are you sure he's straight?"

"Absolutely. He just digs women's clothing."

"What, like ruffled blouses and dresses too?"

"Just panties."

"Honestly, Dee, I don't know if I could handle that. The sex can't be *that* good."

"It is, plus I think part of what's so fun is you get to live like a spy."

"What do you mean?"

"Well, we have to be so careful. He's had other affairs, so he knows what to do to avoid getting caught."

"He's an old pro at this game then?"

"Yes. My God Sharon, you should see what he makes me do."

"What?"

"He arrives at the hotel first. We never show up together, we never leave together." That's something Carrick and I did wrong straight out of the gate.

"What else?" I asked reaching for a notepad.

"He always showers and washes his hair before we leave."

"What else?"

"We never visit the same hotel twice in the same month."

"Sounds like he's very cautious."

"He is. That's what has me worried."

"What are you worried about?"

"Two of my panties are missing."

"No way! Did you leave them at the hotel?"

"No. When the first one went missing, I stripped the bed to find it. It never showed up and then I had to go, so he said he'd look for it."

"What could have happened to it?"

"I think he's taking them."

"Why doesn't he just buy his own?"

"Brace yourself; he only wears panties I've worn."

"Okay, that is just sick, demented, and nasty."

"I know. What I don't know is what he's doing with my undies."

"Wearing 'em for his wife," I said, putting my notepad away.

"I doubt it."

"Are you going to confront him?"

"I don't think so," Dakota sounded despondent.

"You should. Get your underwear back. I hope he isn't stealing the expensive stuff."

"Yes, he is, and now I have two bras without matching panties."

"Are you going to continue seeing him?" The long pause was all the answer I needed.

Dakota's weirdo had my trio of circus freaks beaten by a landslide. I just hoped my next encounter wouldn't be with Bra man. I only wanted one person in the relationship wearing Papillion lace panties and that person was going to be me.

"Would you like to see what he looks like? I have his picture downloaded. I could send it to you."

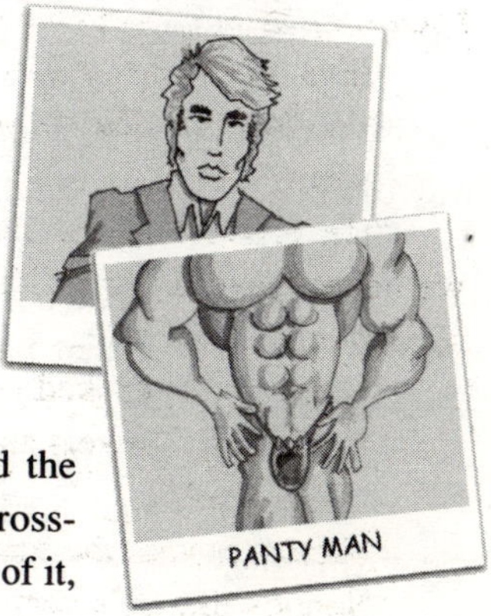

"You do? Does he know? I'm surprised such a paranoid guy would allow his image to be floating around in cyberspace."

"He's not that bad. Although he did make me promise I'd never e-mail his picture, so if I send it to you, you can't show it to anybody else, okay?" What was I going to do, show it around the office? Hey everybody, wanna see a cross-dressing adulterer? Actually, come to think of it, that would certainly make for a memorable casual Friday. "So, do you want to see him?"

"Sure, why not." I wondered which gender clothing he was wearing. I was genuinely curious what a guy who dressed like a woman looked like. I half expected to see Jamie Farr.

"Here he comes." I could hear Dakota hitting keys on her computer. A few seconds later, message from Dakota. I clicked on the attachment. Up popped a picture of Timothy Dalton. But it wasn't Timothy, it was Kevin. He was as close a look-alike as you'd ever want to see. I was speechless. In a word, he was handsome. He wore the same quirky smile Simon had used on us the few times Dakota and I had attempted to make contact. We were never successful at gaining Simon's attention, let alone his affections.

"Well, what do you think?"

"He's gorgeous," I said hitting the print icon. I wanted a hard copy for myself.

"Do you think he looks like Simon?"

"Yeah, but he looks more like Timothy Dalton."

"Wow, I thought so too."

"What are you going to do about your panties?" The picture of Kevin had slipped from the printer. I picked it up. He was really striking.

"Nothing. Do you think I should do anything?"

I was staring at the picture. I found Kevin's eyes totally mesmerizing. How did Dakota always manage to attract such fantastic looking men? Even with a panty fetish, this guy was leaps and bounds ahead of the two I'd attracted. (I am excluding Mike since it's obvious I didn't attract him.)

"Well?" Dakota's voice blared into my thoughts

"Well," I echoed her, "if I were in your shoes, which are actually way too big for me, I would do nothing too."

"Really?"

"Yes, really. If I had a guy who looked like this, not only could he wear my underwear, but hell, I think he could help himself to any garment in my closet."

"Do you honestly feel that way?"

"I think so. What's his body like?"

"Amazing!"

"What about his personality?"

This made Dakota laugh. I laughed too.

"Listen," she said between giggles. "It was an accomplishment just to get his name, rank, and serial number. We don't actually spend a lot of time philosophizing."

"Have you got a picture that shows his body?" The picture Dakota sent was a head shot.

"No, and delete the file I sent, okay?"

"Okay," I said hitting my delete button. No need to save the file when I had a hard copy. Not that I could imagine doing anything other than staring at the image. Kevin's fetish put a whole new twist on the adage, beware of a wolf in sheep's clothing. Especially if the sheep is a she and the clothing is a bikini.

On my way home, I heard a voice call out my name from across the parking lot. A pang of fear went through me as an image of Dinky stalking me came to mind. I turned to see who belonged to the voice. I couldn't believe my eyes.

"Oh my God! Gavin? Is that you?" It was incredible. He'd lost all his extra weight. His face was no longer round; in fact, it was damn sexy. He was about as ripped as a non-fanatical body-builder could be, assuming he was non-fanatical, and a body-builder.

"Gavin, you look amazing!" He had a sheepish expression that denoted he'd gotten used to this reaction from old friends he hadn't seen in a while.

"What the hell happened?"

"I don't know really. I just got in a zone. I got laid off from my job about five years ago. Started drawing unemployment. I had nothing else going on in my life, so I figured, as long as wasn't doing anything, I might as well start working out. I get more and more buff, and that inspired me to eat better. I started consulting with nutritionists and professional trainers and before I knew it, I was a full-blown health and fitness nut. Who would have thought, eh?"

"So other than the getting buff, what else is going on in your life?" I asked, curious if the new look had paid off. Apparently it had.

"Oh my God Sharon, everything. And it's all because of getting buff. About three years ago, I started getting chummy with this guy at my gym and we became workout buddies. Turns out he was this hotshot entrepreneur. He hired me to supervise his network setups.

I've gotten engaged to a really sweet, beautiful girl, who I met just when I was starting to work out, so she's seen me heavy and she liked me anyway."

As Gavin went on about how great his life had become, I started getting that same pang of unease I'd felt when Dakota had told me about Kevin. Gavin finished updating me on his life since we'd parted ways, and told me he was late for a date with his fiancé. We said goodbye and promised to stay in touch. I knew it probably wouldn't happen, I really wanted it to. As Gavin walked away, I was taken aback at how sexy his rear end was. Hard to believe it was the same shapeless, lump that spent four solid years parked on the couch in my living room.

Everybody I ever knew was doing better than I was. And I was totally pissed off about it. I couldn't allow this to eat me up. That wasn't the kind of person I thought I was. Oh sure, I'm shallow and materialistic, I'll be the first to admit that. But envious of others? Unacceptable. I decided right there and then that to feel happy for others, I had to feel happy about myself.

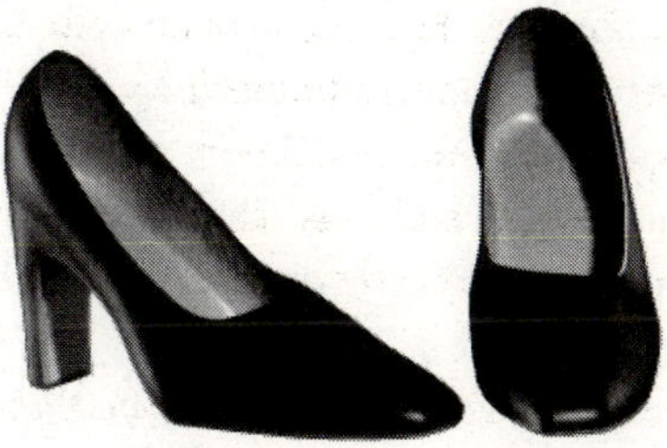

Chapter Six:
Skeletor

After my epiphany, I realized two things. First, I learned from Dakota that it is possible to find love online, you just have to commit yourself to the search. Second, I learned that you have to kiss a lot of frogs before you find one that turns into a prince.

I decided to redouble my efforts in the pursuit of happiness. I was now spending every available minute online, trying to find a reasonable substitute for Dogbiscuit. I was getting scores of messages. At first, this was really exciting because it's always a good thing to be popular. Unfortunately, if I was ever going to read them all, I'd need to hire an assistant. I tried to respond to each message with a personal greeting, but it was very time consuming. A guy who called himself BizzareMan sent a message to me that said, among other things, he was looking for a woman to pamper. Obviously, this is something a lot of men claim they want to do. Apparently it works. Indeed, I have to confess, "pamper" is one of my favorite words. I love everything about that word. All the images it evokes, and the way the letter combination forces your lips into a full pout as the word tumbles from your mouth. Pamper. Doesn't it make you want to purr? After reading that message, I immediately responded. I sent a short note telling him I was very interested in the pampering, and then I asked for specifics. The reason I asked for specifics is because I once spent half an hour instant messaging another man who, as it turned out, had a bizarre definition of "pamper".

BizzareMan: *Do you want to be pampered?*

SharonSharalike: *Sure.*

BizzareMan: *What would you like, a massage or a foot rub?*

SharonSharalike: *Why do I have to choose? Can't I have both?*

BizzareMan: *lol. You are greedy aren't you?*

SharonSharalike: *I am not greedy; I just like to be pampered.*

BizzareMan: *Okay, sweetie, you get both.*

SharonSharalike: *I'd like to have those services at the Still Water Spa, please and thank you.*

BizzareMan: *No, I'm going to do them.*

SharonSharalike: *Oh, do you work at the Elm?*

BizzareMan: *No I don't work at a spa. But I love to pamper.*

SharonSharalike: *Have you got any sort of formal training in foot rubbing?*

BizzareMan: *No, but I have a strong desire to please. Does that count?*

SharonSharalike: *Let me get this straight, you aren't a trained masseuse.*

BizzareMan: *That's right. But I love to pamper.*

SharonSharalike: *Well, if you have no skills, don't you think you should send me to a professional?*

BizzareMan: *I have skills.*

SharonSharalike: *You just admitted that you don't have formal training!*

BizzareMan: *I don't need training to rub your feet.*

SharonSharalike: *Yes, you do. If you are really interested in pampering me, and you don't want to send me to a spa, and you want to involve my feet, what about a gift certificate to Cole Hann?*

BizzareMan: *I said pamper, not take you on a shopping spree.*

SharonSharalike: *Aren't they the same thing?*

BizzareMan: *Not where I come from.*

SharonSharalike: *When I think of pampering, I think of mornings spent at the spa, afternoons shopping on Bloor Street, dinner at a four star, and a night at the Sutton Place.*

BizzareMan: *Sounds like you're looking for a man with deep pockets.*

SharonSharalike: *Actually, I am looking for a man who knows the difference between pampering a lady and indulging in a foot fetish.*

After that I signed off. You can see how a single instant message session, and writing a couple of e-mails, can consume a lot of time. As a result, I'm not doing a very good job keeping up with my correspondence. This, of course, is beginning to tick some men off. I've received a few nasty ratings on my profile report card. The website has a system whereby people who communicate with you can leave their opinion of you in the form of either a smile or a frown, based on whether or not they liked the interaction. Right now, I have a surplus of frowns, while my smiles seem to be dwindling at an alarming rate. How am I going to turn things around? Perhaps I should put a little note on my profile that says something like: *Due to my recent surge in popularity, it may take some time for me to respond to your message. Please allow two weeks for a reply, your notes are important to me*. That might help placate some of the eager beavers.

I've recently been devoting my Internet hours to a guy called Schooner. I love that name, not just because it conjures images of being out on the Pacific Ocean, sailing around with a bottle of Perrier and an orange life preserver. No, I think of being in university and living on campus. Schooner was my favorite beer during my college years. Every pubcrawl, pubnight, and St. Patrick's Day (when I did venture from my room) was accompanied by a tall glass of Schooner, and a basket of pretzels.

The first time I received a message from Schooner, my heart actually skipped a beat, did a summersault and landed in my throat. Reading that name overwhelmed me with a tidal wave of forgotten (suppressed?) memories. I could see myself dancing at the campus club, to music by Dead or Alive, until my head was spinning, just like the record, baby, around, and around. Before my glasses flew off my face, the DJ mercifully started playing something by Adam Ant. Oh, the eighties! Remember how cool it was for men to wear makeup and puff their hair up like those troll dolls? Those were the good times. I should have drunk more, and read less. I sometimes wish I'd recall fewer useless details from that glorious time when parachute pants were a sign of hip, cutting-edge fashion sense.

I can attribute my excellent memory to the fact that I was, almost always, the designated driver, although no one I knew had a car. My job was to help everyone else find the toilet, their jacket, or the way home. With such memories, is it any wonder I felt an immediate connection to Schooner, even if it was just a nostalgic response to the name?

Right from the start, I could tell Schooner was different from the other men I'd met online. Unlike other guys, he seemed to want to know me, not my bra size. Another thing I liked about him was that he took the time to write long, thoughtful messages. Each message ended with an endearing little question. What are the issues that concern you? Was the question attached to the first message he ever sent me. Isn't it nice that he wanted to know what I cared about? That is so sweet. I sent back a message with the list of things that are real issues for me:

Dry skin

Fine lines and wrinkles

How to get my French manicure to last longer than five days!

Split ends

Pantyhose that run the first time you wear them

Panties that want to be thongs but aren't! (So uncomfortable!)

Schooner wrote me back almost immediately with his list. When I read his concerns, all I could think was, *oops*. I had no idea that by concerns he meant humanitarian efforts. On his list were things like:

Assisting refugees from Bosnia

Famine relief in the Sudan

The legalization of marijuana for the terminally ill

I should have written stuff like that too. There are so many global issues that concern me. For example, that channel that always shows poor starving children really leaves me depressed. And that's not all. I also intend to donate blood someday... as soon as the Red Cross provides a proper recovery meal instead of two stale sugar cookies and half a Dixie cup of diluted orange juice. It's just not right to offer such a lame snack when someone has parted with an entire liter of blood. I think, a cheeseburger, fries, and a shake are in order.

At least Schooner didn't think badly of me after he'd read my list. I must have looked like a self-absorbed twit. However, since he was still talking to me, I was sure he had the good sense to realize that there's a little bit of Mother Theresa in all of us. But I was having difficulty locating the little bit that's in me. I'm sure it'll turn up one of these days.

I told Schooner to send me his phone number in his next e-mail. This was the second time I had to ask a man. I was hoping he'd send me his number soon so we could talk while I was at work. Yes, I know I wasn't going to make personal calls at work any more, but hey, you know how it is. I still needed to have sex. It was August and I was getting desperate. I'd taped Dinky's cell number to the side of my monitor. It was folded so no one could read it. On the outside flap I printed: *Use only in the case of emergency!*

Dinky's number was my motivation to continue with my quest to find a suitable surrogate for Dogbiscuit. Each night, after the children went to bed, I logged onto MadAsh for a few hours. Even though I was deep in what felt like political negotiations with Schooner, I kept other options open.

Schooner sent me an instant message indicating he wanted to meet me, but only on his terms. He didn't want to do coffee, because he didn't feel that would give us enough time to get to know each other. He didn't want to do lunch, because the lunch crowd was usually noisy, and service tended to be negligent. Schooner was convinced that fine restaurants, those which open for lunch, want to rush you out so they can enjoy a siesta before preparing for the dinner crowd.

I sent him an instant message that said: *Perhaps we should have dinner together.*

Normally I like a quick meeting. Coffee is my preference. It's quick and relatively painless. If the date begins to sour, you can exit fast. Lunch and dinner require more time, and if you aren't getting along, there are so many courses to sit through. I think Schooner was considering this as well. After a while, he wrote: *Sometimes the service can be really slow.*

The rest of the conversation went like this:

SharonSharalike: *Tell me about it. Once I had to wait twenty-five minutes for a salad. What could possibly account for such a long wait?*

Schooner: *Maybe they were picking the tomatoes.*

SharonSharalike: *I don't know about that. The salad looked like it came out of a Ready Mix bag.*

Schooner: *I like those salads.*

SharonSharalike: *Me too, but it doesn't take twenty-five minutes to make it.*

Schooner: *Well, the other thing I hate are the prices.* Uh-oh. Red alert, all systems stand by, there could be a cheapo on the line.

SharonSharalike: *What about the prices?* I typed cautiously.

I hoped Schooner wasn't the kind of guy who liked to order two appetizers in place of one entree.

Schooner: *I've had some experiences in which I wasn't getting value for my money.*

SharonSharalike: *Ironically, I stopped associating value with eating when I started ordering McValue meals.*

Schooner: *lol. Value is still important. I want a fair shake every time I make a purchase.*

Schooner and Dogbiscuit would enjoy each other. I expected Schooner to launch into a lecture about my spending habits.

Schooner: *I think sometimes the prices are too high and the decor too meager.*

SharonSharalike: *In some restaurants, the decor is so poorly coordinated you need an antacid just to get through the appetizer.*

Although I had vowed to become a kinder, gentler Sharon, Schooner was making it hard for me. After we had critiqued just about every restaurant in the city, he asked if I was available on Friday. Even though I knew I was totally free, I told him I'd have to check my calendar and get back to him. I promised to let him know by Wednesday.

I was reluctant to commit myself to a meeting, because I'd started having a few misgivings about Schooner. There was something about him that was starting to irritate me, and considering I'd never met him, this seemed a bit weird. I hadn't even talked to him on the phone. I didn't want to dump him just yet, because I loved the questions in his messages. The night before, he'd asked me what three things I'd bring with me if I were stranded on a desert island. I said butter, a nail file, and *Cosmo*. Of course he had to tell me what he'd bring, although I knew better than to ask. Schooner said he'd bring a Swiss Army knife, because you can do just about anything with it, Gandhi would tag along, because of his teachings. The third item would be me, for the same reason as the knife. Wasn't that sweet? Of course if I'd known I could bring dead people, I would have brought Vidal Sasoon and left *Cosmopolitan* at the newsstand. *Cosmo* just has pictures of great hair styles; Vidal could actually give me one. Just because you're marooned, it's no reason to let your looks go to Hell.

That Tuesday, I received a message from Schooner saying he'd made reservations for Friday. When I heard this, I was of two minds. Part of me wanted to be upset because I had yet to confirm that I was available; the other part of me was jumping for joy. The reservations were for Scaramouch, an upscale restaurant on a hill overlooking downtown. Schooner finally sent his cell number. I called him as soon as I finished reading his e-mail, and no, I didn't wait for my lunch break.

"Hello?" Deep sexy voice. Good sign.

"Hello. Schooner?"

"Yes?" Next came some throat clearing, and a cough.

I sent up a silent prayer: *Please don't let him be the nervous type.*

"It's me, Sharon Sharalike," I said.

"Hello, Sharon," he said. Now that he'd cleared his throat, his voice wasn't so deep.

"I'm sorry, I don't know your name," I said expectantly.

"Steve," he said. His voice was deep again. What was going on with him? Puberty?

"Hi Steve," I said.

"How are you Sharon?"

"Good thanks," I replied.

"Great, I'm doing well too."

Did I ask how he was? No, so why was he telling me?

"I got your message a little while ago," I said trying to move things along.

"Good, and...?"

"And I'm really impressed. Scaramouch. Wow," I said enthusiastically.

"Are you free?" How come I can never answer this guy's questions correctly?

"Yes, of course I am."

"Before, you indicated you might not be able to make it."

Well, that was before I knew where you were planning to take me. Duh!

"Yes well, fortunately, I will be able to see you on Friday."

"Excellent," he said. His voice was high pitched again. It seemed to squeak on words with more than three syllables.

"Okay, so I'll drop you a message then."

"Please do. Let me know what you're wearing."

"Right now?" I asked, totally shocked. He laughed, I didn't.

"No, what you'll be wearing on Friday." More laughing. A nice low sound.

"Okay, bye," I said, wanting to hang up fast.

"Thanks for calling."

"It was a pleasure," I said.

"Indeed." The way he said that one word sent shivers up and down my arms. "Indeed" only has two syllables, so Schooner/Steve's voice didn't crack or squeak. *Au contraire*, it was deep and velvety smooth like chocolate. I hung up, pushed my swivel chair back and used my feet to spin around a few times.

"This is not an amusement park, and your chair is not a Merry-Go-Round." I dropped my right foot to the floor and ground to an abrupt halt. I sat up straight and looked around. Ralph was hanging over the cubicle partition looking at me. I smiled, gave him the finger and went back to work. Not "work" work. I went back to work thinking about Friday and making plans. I was definitely going to have to find time to shop.

The next morning, I left the house early and headed off to my favorite mall. I thought I could spend my time more efficiently there than on Bloor Street. At the mall you don't have to deal with things like stairs and doors, unless, of course, you're trying to get in when the sales girls are locking up for the night.

Dakota has annoyed more than a few sales people by slipping through the closing doors. Even I won't stoop to rolling under the cage doors when there's only a few shopping moments left. Dakota could single-handedly make a twenty-four-hour mall a lucrative venture. I'll bet the retail sector would thrive if there was a twenty-four-hour mall. I must remember to mention that to Schooner, because that's a global issue that concerns me. Longer shopping hours would be a real shot in the arm for business. That would help all sorts of industries. The next time Dogbiscuit tells me I buy too much, I'll tell him I'm not shopping, I'm helping to boost the economy.

The first store I entered had naked mannequins in their display window. Good, that always meant a sale was either eminent or in progress. I headed to the back of the store toward the sales rack. When I was younger, I never did that. I'd always start at the front and ease my way over to sale items with lots of high priced merchandise dangling from my arms. Now I don't care if the world knows I shop principally for bargains. I think it makes sense. Thanks to Dogbiscuit's lack of generosity, I only have a few fashion dollars to spend and they stretch farther over discounted items than regular priced items.

I carefully went through the sales rack, but I didn't find anything I liked. Everything looked like Salvation Army cast-offs. Did they import stuff especially for the sale rack? None of the items looked like they'd ever been regular priced. Disgusted, I moved over to the neatly stacked, folded sweaters. A sales girl moved in on me. She was shadowing my every move. I read her nametag, Kimberly, and then tried to put some space between us. It was a big store, couldn't she fold sweaters near the front? One good thing about looking through red-tagged merchandise is that the sales girls leave you alone to bargain-hunt in peace.

"These just came in," Kimberly said, touching the pile of sweaters like she was auditioning to be one of Barker's beauties on *The Price Is Right*.

"Good," I said, trying to move away from her. Is it really necessary for you to stand so close to me? It was bad enough I could read her name tag without squinting, but now I could also see that she hadn't bothered to blend her eye shadow at the corners of her eyes. They were a very pretty blue though.

"Are you looking for anything special?"

"Yes, I am."

"Something like this?" Kimberly held up a thin cashmere sweater in baby blue.

"That's beautiful, but it's not what I'm looking for."

"Well, can you describe it?"

"Six feet or taller, dark hair, light eyes, swarthy complexion."

"What?" Kimberly laughed like a girl. She was probably still in her teens.

"I could also use a black skirt with a swing."

"Oh, I know just the thing." She ran nosily across the hardwood floor, grabbed a dark garment off a rack, and came running back to me, beaming.

"What do you think?"

Well, it was black, and it was a skirt. But it didn't have any type of swing. I had plenty of skirts like the one Kimberly held up. What I wanted was one that flowed around my body, and bounced when I walked.

I smiled at her. "It's great, but it doesn't really move, does it?"

"Well, no, but check out how great it looks with this," Kimberly darted off again. The outfit she put together was actually very nice. The skirt was short, black and peppy. The top was a body-hugging, tank with a black and white Japanese art pattern. I loved it. However, was it the right sort of thing for Scaramouch?

"I like this," I told Kimberly, "but have you got anything more formal?"

"Uh-mmmm." Kimberly's cute face was scrunched up as she tried to think. I had to help her out before her head exploded.

"Any long skirts?"

"What about a dress?"

"That might work," I said hopeful. Kimberly galloped to the front of the store. She pulled out a dress and I almost fainted, it was that gorgeous.

"There's only a size two left." She held up what looked like half a dress on a wooden hanger. On my really, really, good days, I'm a size four. Getting into a size two might be possible with some designers. But the dress Kim held was so minuscule it looked too small to be a tea cozy.

"I'm sorry about the size," Kim said. For a moment it looked like she was going to return it to the rack.

"That's okay," I said, quickly taking the hanger from her. "I'm sure it will fit." I couldn't leave the store without it. I'd cut my own thighs off if I had to.

"Do you want to try it on?"

"Absolutely," I said admiring the shear fabric. I followed

Kimberly to the back of the store. The dress was obviously by the same designer as the tank top I'd admired; it's look was reminiscent of Japanese art. I held the dress against my body so I could see where the hem would fall. The dress was cut in an A-line, so its skirt flowed out from the waist, and swayed gently above my knees. That was exactly the look I'd been after with the skirt.

"There you go." Kimberly pushed open the door of a changing room.

"Thank you," I said, stepping inside. I closed the door and latched it. I slipped my clothes off quickly. When I reached for the dress, the garment tags brushed against my arm. I hadn't even looked at the price. I figured the dress was around $300, and checked to confirm my guess. I had to blink several times when I caught sight of the price. How could a little wisp of a dress in a mall store cost so damn much? I checked the price tag again. I stood absolutely still in my Calvin Klein white cotton bikini panties. I wasn't sure whether I should try on a dress that expensive, or whether I should throw in the towel and try another store.

"How is it?"

"I'm not in it yet," I said, knowing I sounded flabbergasted. Fuck, now Kim was going to think it was too small. I had to try on the overpriced scrap of fabric, just to show her I know my own dress size.

I put on the dress and stepped out.

"Wow!" Kim covered her face with her hands. I moved to the three-way mirror. Wow, indeed. The dress looked like it was cut right on my body. It flowed over every dip, curve, and groove. I looked stunning.

"You are so tiny," Kim said, putting her hands on her own generous hips.

"I've been starving myself," I told her, proud that my efforts had reduced me to a size two. I made a mental note to go to McDonald's and celebrate.

I decided to buy the dress because it was just too beautiful to pass up. And anyway, I thought I deserved a reward for getting skinny. Sex would have been better, but I hadn't reached the state of liberation that would allow me to purchase sex as a reward. Kimberly packaged my dress with lots of tissue, then placed it in a fabric bag, which I guess explains why that store was so expensive. I should have left the mall with my dress, but I still had an hour and twenty-five minutes before work. I had plenty of time for a quick look around.

I headed straight for William & Sonoma. I spent my time there looking at martini glasses and shakers. Next, I looked at kitchen gadgets. It's too bad I've never taken an interest in cooking. Thank God my kids love hot dogs and Kraft Dinner so much. I picked up a saucepan. It was so heavy, I almost couldn't get it off the counter. With cookware like this, I could develop my biceps just making spaghetti twice a week. I left William & Sonoma after promising the sales clerk I'd return for the martini shaker.

I took a sharp right into Pottery Barn for Kids. I wanted to gasp at the over-priced teddy bears and crib toys. There was a bin with some rag dolls. I had purchased one for Mackenzie in March. The dolls were on sale for half of what I'd paid. I hate it when that happens. I was so put off, I made a U-turn out of the store.

I checked my watch to see how many more stores I could visit. I almost yelped out loud. Where had all the time gone? I had only fifteen minutes to get to work. I started to walk as quickly as I could toward the exit. It took me a full twelve minutes to get out of the mall and another three minutes to locate my car. I was late for work before I even got onto to the road heading south. When I arrived at the office, Ralph greeted me with a "Tsk, tsk, tsk". I used to blame my tardiness on the subway system. Sometimes it was an ill passenger, other times it was malfunctioning doors on one of the cars. That was before I drove my own car to work. Now, I don't make any apologies, I just try to switch the subject.

"Hey Ralph, you look good today. New tie?" Ralph looked down at his chest instead of at the office wall clock. "Things going well with Victoria?"

"Veronica," he corrected, "and yes, things are good. She's coming over tonight."

"Whatcha' cooking," I asked, scooting into my desk and removing items from my "Do Immediately" file.

"Nothing, she's coming over for drinks."

"Oh you are a smart one, aren't you, Ralph." I gave him a wink.

"What are you talking about?"

"Don't play dumb with me. I know that maneuver. You're going to juice her up to loosen her up."

"Sharon, we're having drinks on my patio."

"Followed by a game of Hide and Seek, Ring Around the Rosie, or What Time Is It Mr. Wolf?"

"Don't you ever stop thinking about sex?"

"Ralph, shame on you! Those are indoor party games. Incidentally, no, I never stop thinking about sex, do you?"

"Of course I do. There's more to life than sex."

"Yes, there's also shopping. I am totally into S & S."

"Talk to you later," Ralph started moving away.

"Wait, wait, Ralph listen, if your girlfriend likes Ring Around the Rosie, try playing Pop Goes the Weasel. She'll love it!"

"Sharon, you're so twisted." Ralph moved away from my desk fast and stayed away for the rest of the week.

On Friday, I was so excited I decided to skip work. I knew if I went in, I would just spend the day fantasizing about the night. Instead, I could make really good use of my time by having a manicure. I stayed in bed waiting for Dogbiscuit to leave for work, so I could begin my day of leisure by calling in sick.

"Sharon, are you awake?" Dogbiscuit asked.

"No," I said trying to sound sleepy. I was wide awake. I could have added an entire row of sums, my brain was so clear.

"What the devil was wrong with you last night?"

"Worms," I said.

"Well, go see a doctor for heaven's sake. I can't sleep in the same bed with a Mexican jumping bean. Another night like that and I'm going to get you your own bed."

"Will it come with its own apartment?"

"I think you should avoid drinking coffee after dinner."

"I don't drink coffee!" I shouted sitting up. "You drink coffee after dinner. Don't you know anything about me?"

"I know that you're going to be sleeping in the guest room very soon if you don't look after your problem." I couldn't believe Dogbiscuit was threatening me. All I could think was, why didn't I think of that sooner? I'd enjoy the privacy and peace of the guest room. I'd move in on Saturday. Dogbiscuit left and I called in sick. I was free to get on with my rendezvous with Schooner.

I arrived at the restaurant at five minutes after eight. I was so proud of myself, because I am usually ten to fifteen minutes late.

The maitre d' addressed me with a courteous nod.

"Reservations?" I knew Schooner had made reservations but I didn't know his last name,

"I'm here to meet someone," I said.

"Name?"

"Steve..."

"Oh, right this way, Madame." Wow, he knew Schooner by his first name. That was impressive. I followed the maitre d' to a table overlooking the city. Such a spectacular view. There was a man in a dark suit seated with his back to us. The maitre d' headed straight for him. As we approached the broad-shouldered mystery man, he turned abruptly to face us. He smiled and stood.

You know that old adage "You can never be too rich or too thin?" Well the "thin" part doesn't apply to men. Men can be too thin. When I looked at Schooner, it was like looking into the face of He-Man's mortal enemy, Skeletor. He was so thin, his face looked like a skull covered in peach toned rice paper.

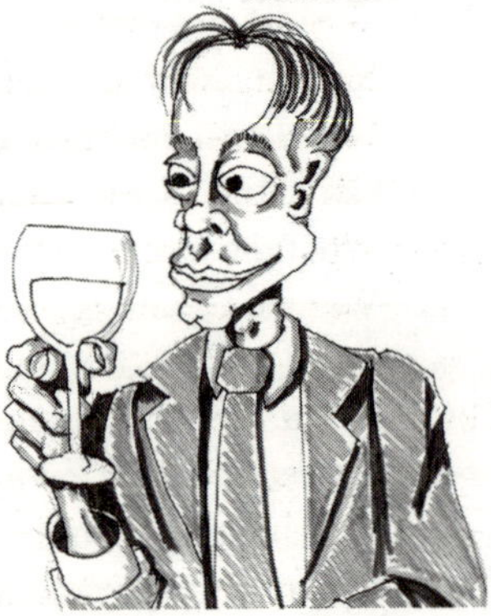

"Sharon," the deep voice rang out.

"Hello, Steve," I held out my hand. He took it and pulled me toward his hollow chest for a hug. He was surprisingly strong.

"Sit down," he said. That should've been an invitation, but it came out like a command. I quickly took the seat held out by the maitre d'. I looked over at Skeletor. He was addressing the maitre d'.

"We'll take our wine now, thank you." The man made a dignified nod, but then scurried off like he, too, feared the dark lord.

"You are stunning. What a gorgeous dress."

I brought my eyes back to Skeletor. "Thank you, Steve" I said, feeling pleased. He hadn't committed any of the technical errors of his predecessors. Perfect greeting, followed by sincere sounding compliment. What more could I ask for? Maybe a guy who didn't look like Unicef's poster boy.

"I've ordered a very fruity Muscat. You will enjoy it. Have a look at the menu."

You will enjoy it? Is that a recommendation or an order? I picked up the heavy menu, and Skeletor did the same. I read through the entrees, then doubled backed to the appetizers. After that, I fast-forwarded to the desserts. I almost always select a chicken dish when I dine out. I peeked over the top of my menu. Skeletor was reading his like the *Sunday Times*. Did we have the same menu?

"Have you made any selections?" he asked.

"Yes," I said, lowering my menu. I closed it and placed it on the table.

"Pick that up, I want to point out some things to you." I jumped, and did as he said. His voice was sharp and stern. He sounded like a drill sergeant.

"Were you ever in the military, Steve?"

"Uh-uh," he laughed. It was a weird sound. Not the diabolical laugh of a deranged scientist, but almost like a cough. "No, does that disappoint you?"

"No," I said, waiting for him to tell me what I should be looking at.

"What do you enjoy?" he asked.

"Reading, running, and shopping."

"I meant as a main course."

"Oh," I said feeling the heat rise to my face. Did he have to sound so smug and condescending?

"The pasta here is exceptional. The swordfish is also beautifully prepared. I've had the salmon once or twice, and it, too, is worthy of even the most discerning palates."

"I was going to have the grilled chicken in the mango orange glaze." Uh-oh, did I say something wrong? His eyes looked like they were about to pop right out of their sockets.

"You really shouldn't eat meat."

"Tonight, or ever?"

"Ever. It takes years to digest. Years."

"All right," I said, raising my menu to my face. This guy was whacked. I wonder if I could slip into the washroom and escape through an open window? I looked over my right shoulder in the direction of the washrooms.

"May I recommend something?"

"Certainly," I returned my attention to the menu.

"Try the swordfish." If that was a recommendation, I didn't want to hear what an order sounded like.

"Okay," I said agreeably, although fish was the last thing I felt like eating. With any luck I could "Indiana Jones" my way out of the restaurant before the entree arrived. The chandelier in the middle of the room looked pretty sturdy. All I needed was a lasso. I glanced around the room, first to my left, then to my right. Everyone looked like they were having a lovely time, while I was stuck with Skeletor. Where was He-Man when you needed him?

"Beautiful view tonight." So far he'd kept his words restricted to two syllables, so his voice remained deep and evenly pitched. When he spoke, his jaw dropped up and down like a hand puppet's. He was beginning to creep me out.

The windows to my left revealed a breath-taking view of the city. The curtains, which covered the floor-to-ceiling windows, were held back by gold ropes. All I had to do was untie one, swing it over my head, latch it onto the chandelier, and swing like Tarzan out the front doors. I could do it, I thought.

"Here we go," I looked over at Skeletor, who was looking at a waiter approaching our table with a bottle of wine. The waiter presented him the bottle. A curt nod let the waiter know the offering was acceptable, so he opened the bottle deftly, and poured a small amount into a wine glass. Skeletor tipped his glass, held it up and actually checked for sediment. Then, much to my horror, he took a sip and gargled the wine like Scope. I could hear him. I looked at the waiter but he was the model of professionalism with an impassive expression on his face. I looked around at the other diners. No one else was put off by the gargling. But then, they didn't seem the least bit interested that I was dining with the arch nemesis of the Master of the Universe. When I returned my gaze to the table, the waiter was pouring the wine into my glass. He filled Skeletor's glass and placed the bottle in the ice bucket beside the table.

"May I take your orders?" he asked, dispassionately.

"Yes, the lady will have the swordfish, and I will have salmon."

"Very good, sir," the waiter made a little bow and left with the menus.

"A toast." Skeletor held up his wine glass. "Here's to you, the brightest star tonight." Well, that was very nice. I could drink to that.

"Cheers," I said, clinking my glass against his. His bony fingers looked like they'd never seen the light of day. I took a sip. It was very nice wine, with a slight pineapple flavor.

"Is it to your liking?"

"Oh, it's very good. It would be great with roast chicken." Uh-oh, I forgot he doesn't eat meat. "Sorry," I added quickly.

"You're fixated on meat aren't you?"

"No, I wouldn't say that. I eat meat because I'm at the top of the food chain."

"Really?"

"Yes, and besides it tastes good."

"So, you eat anything that tastes good?" His voice dripped with disdain.

"Sure, if it's not fattening."

"Would you eat me, if I tasted good?"

"I prefer cows and chickens."

"I find the senseless killing of animals appalling. There's plenty for us to eat without resorting to animal killing." Could this get any worse? At least back in college, when Gavin was raving along these lines, I never had to pay any heed. Skeletor made compliance downright mandatory.

"Killing cows isn't really senseless killing; it's economical." I couldn't believe I was still trying to debate this rationally.

"How's that?" he asked, not prepared to agree with the answer.

"We use every single part of that animal. We consume the meat, and we tan the hides to create clothing, purses and stuff."

"I suppose you have a closet full of leather clothing, purses, and shoes."

"Yes, but I also have a vegan jacket."

"A vegan jacket? Never heard of such a thing."

"It's made from vegetarians. Ha ha ha." Skeletor's face was stone cold. I laughed again anyway, and the more I laughed, the more Skeletor frowned.

"Excuse me, Steve," I said, "I suddenly have a craving for a double cheeseburger and a chocolate shake." I stood up, drained my wine glass, took a final look out the window at the gorgeous view. And walked away from the table and out the door without a single backward glance.

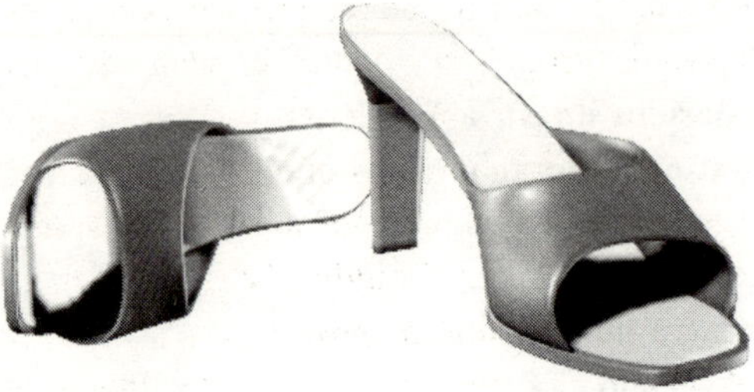

Chapter Seven:
Mr. Bombastic

It's amazing to me how little married men know about dating. Quite frankly, I don't understand. The same rules applied when they were single. Perhaps marriage has caused their brains to atrophy. When I think about the men I've met on Ashley Madison, all four seem woefully uninformed about the dos and don'ts of dating. After years of living happily, or otherwise, in the sanctity of marriage, it isn't easy to re-enter the dating game, particularly if you remain attached, and your new partner is likewise.

I think the standards of practice are a little more stringent when men date married women, because we're far less forgiving than our single counterparts. I figure if a man has been married or lived with a woman, he should know how to dress, how to greet me, and where to take me on our first, second, and even third date, should things progress blissfully towards the Hilton. A married man should know what to do to impress a woman. By that I don't mean indulging in a bring and brag session. Please don't bring me to your car so you can go on and on about it. I admit, I enjoy a posh ride in a really swank automobile. But a high status car alone doesn't make a man, it just makes driving with him more comfortable. What usually impresses me is a man who's well spoken, well dressed, and well mannered. I still haven't met a man who can walk away with an A in all three categories.

Mike, for example, showed up in pants so short I thought he was wearing GAP Capri's. Was he expecting a flood? Did he think he might have to wade through six inches of water to get to me? Had Mike bothered to invest in a full-length mirror, I could have been spared several excruciating moments of embarrassment. As it was, the three minutes he spent walking me to my car felt like a month-long journey to Mecca. Good looks shouldn't be offered as a substitute for good grooming and clothes that fit properly.

While I'm on this subject, there was one other thing that got on my nerves. It happened with both Elephant Man and Dinky. They greeted me like I was an appetizer they hadn't ordered. I don't quite understand how that happens. Doesn't everyone realize that you only get one chance at a first impression?

Elephant Man approached me right after that guy who looked like Brian Adams. His name was Allen I think. No, no it was Andrew. Yes, Andrew. I rather like that name. I should take a detour through Chapters one morning to see if he's around. I still remember how he mellowed me with that simple, lovely compliment.

That morning, I had it going on. I looked "soda-licious." Which is not how I normally appear before noon. Ironically, Elephant Man didn't come right over and scoop me up. No, instead he cowered somewhere between the stacks of *Good Housekeeping* and *Popular Mechanics*. I wonder what Elephant Man would have done if I'd walked out of Chapters with Andrew in tow. He probably would've complained to someone else that Sharon Sharalike stood him up. It's fortunate for Elephant Man that I'm only able to focus on meeting one guy at a time. Otherwise, Andrew's fast-talking flattery and seize-the-moment bravado, could have put Elephant Man out of the game permanently. Not that it mattered, since his own big head sidelined him.

Rounding out the top three losers was Dinky. He greeted me with an awkward handshake, as if he was a mortgage broker and I was a client who had Park Avenue dreams and a Bronx budget. I would have preferred a hug. Dinky and I spent weeks talking on the phone before we met for lunch. A hug would've been appropriate, and a welcome reprieve from my normally unaffectionate routine. The handshake only served to set up a wall of formality between us, which took most of the lunch hour, and incredible dexterity on my part, to surmount.

I wish men would pick up their cues from a woman's body language. Don't get me wrong. A warm handshake is great, especially at church. Hugs, on the other hand, have a way of making you feel connected and appreciated. For that reason alone, I'll take a hug any time, followed by a nice comment about my appearance. It takes days to prepare for a date, and Dinky and Elephant Man didn't make a single memorable comment about my appearance. Someone should explain to them that flattery can get you all the things diamonds can, without depleting your bank account. Unless you look like Skeletor.

Skeletor was close to being the perfect guy. Perfect, that is, if you ignored that he was so thin he looked like a partially assembled IKEA coat rack. Skeletor was right on the money in so many ways, but then he had to spoil it with his dictator routine. Does his wife put up with that Mussolini act? If I couldn't stand him after forty-five minutes, how could any woman possibly endure twenty years of marriage? That's how long he said he'd been married. I should have asked him how many wives he'd had in that time.

The thing that bugged me the most about Skeletor was his attempt to convert me into a herbivore. I love a good salad too, but enough is enough. I'm not a bloody rabbit. I need to eat a steak once in a while. And there's nothing wrong with chicken. It's a staple of the North American diet. Lest we forget, Colonel Sanders died a multi-millionaire. Let Skeletor chew on that drumstick. The one thing I am loath to confess is that I did like the way Skeletor took matters into his own hands. That macho, take-charge attitude gets me every time. I mean, it makes me feel so, dare I say it, pampered, to have a man order my wine and select my meal. But why couldn't he have picked the Mango Chicken?

Some men are so wishy-washy, always differing to the woman's choice, the woman's desires. It's not chivalrous, as one instant messenger claimed. I think it's simply passing the buck. I want a man who knows what he's all about. Not the Dogbiscuit variety who answers every question with "I dunno, you decide." It's sort of sexy to have all the major decisions made before the girl arrives, don't you think? Kudos to Skeletor for selecting such a gorgeous wine. I wanted to take it with me when I got up to leave, but I couldn't think of a way to get out of the restaurant with it. In the end, I just settled for draining my wine glass. I should have drunk his too. God knows he didn't need the alcohol. He already looked like a dehydrated rutabaga. How does anyone get that thin? I bet he has lists and lists of foods he doesn't eat.

After my dating debacle with Skeletor, I drove straight to the liquor store. I wasn't planning on drowning myself in a bottle of Vodka, although the thought was compelling. Instead, my goal was to grab another bottle of the lovely wine that should have accompanied my chicken dinner. I arrived at the liquor store six minutes before it closed. There's nothing like a five speed-transmission, BMW engineering, and desperation, to maneuver you through Friday night traffic. Dakota would have been proud of me. Dakota. I wondered how she and Kevin were doing. I decided to get something to drink and head over to her place and bury the hatchet. It should be pretty easy since she didn't even know there was a hatchet. When I walked in through the sliding doors, the cashier nearest the doors turned and gave me a nasty look. I smiled.

"You're still open, right?" I asked cheerfully.

"Yeah, for another five minutes," was the sour reply. I was certain I only needed three minutes. I knew it was an Ontario wine, and I knew it was a Muscat. Unfortunately, I never got a good look at the label. I thought I'd be able to identify it by the color and shape of the bottle, but you know what? No matter how distinctive a bottle looks on your table, in the liquor store, one bottle looks pretty much the same as any other. I knew the clock was ticking, and even though there were quite a few other shoppers in the store, I felt under the gun.

"Oh, to hell with it," I muttered under my breath. I would send Skeletor an e-mail requesting the name of the wine and apologizing for not wanting to see him again. Ever.

I grabbed a blush from the wine cooler. It was a bottle of Ernest & Julio Gallo, my tried and true brand. You can always depend on them for a good drink. No frills, but at least I was certain I wasn't going to end up with another bottle of cooking wine.

"How fast was that?" I asked the same sour attendant.

"I'm impressed," he said smiling. "I like a lady who knows what she wants."

"Funny, I was just thinking the same thing about men."

In my car, I debated between driving to Dakota's place as planned and just going home. If I went home, and if Dogbiscuit noticed my dress, there was a good chance we'd get into a fight. I decided to stick with Dakota's place. With just a tiny bit of luck, she'd be home. I drove to her condo with my fingers crossed.

The weather had become quite pleasant and by the time I arrived at Dakota's place, the gardens were lit up with little patio lights that looked like Chinese lanterns. I followed them up the walkway that led to four sets of glass doors. The doors were tinted a smoky brown that looked spectacular against the brass door fittings. I entered the building and headed straight for the concierge's desk.

It was the same guy who'd been on duty the night Dakota and I stumbled in with our plan to join Ashley Madison.

"Good evening," he said. His face lit up with recognition when I reached his desk. I leaned onto the round cherry wood console. The console was covered with six screens and enough buttons to launch him into orbit.

"Hi," I said, smiling wildly at the thought of him in zero gravity. Come to think of it, his desk did look a bit like Kazoo's spaceship. "Dakota Montgomery, please." I waited as he buzzed her. I've never seen anyone leave or enter Dakota's building. But I knew there were some high rollers on the top floors. Rich people must spend a lot of time away from their homes. I heard the concierge talking. That was a good sign.

"Ms. Montgomery is expecting you."

"Great, thank you very much." The concierge rounded his desk, leaving his jacket on the chair. He was tall, with broad shoulders and a narrow waist. He had a nice, flat stomach. Such a good physique for a guy who sits all day. Maybe he was sucking in his gut. I followed him to the elevators and he summoned the elevator for me. When the doors opened, he leaned in and pressed Dakota's floor so I could continue to clutch my purse with one hand, and the cold wine bottle with the other. I'm sure I had the look of a desperate woman. When the elevator doors opened, Dakota was waiting for me. Instead of allowing me to get out, she got in.

"Kal's home."

"Fuck," I said.

"Maybe I can send him out."

"Good idea, tell him I need tampons and a pregnancy test."

"You idiot, those are mutually exclusive items."

"Right, right." I said. We both giggled like schoolgirls. "Tell him I need the tampons and you need the pregnancy test," I shot back in a stroke of brilliance.

"Oh boy, don't even joke about a thing like that."

"Dakota, you're not…?" I felt my stomach muscles contract. If there was one person on the planet who shouldn't have children, it was Dakota. She can't even look after plants.

"Don't worry," she said leading me from the elevator, "I'm not."

"Good," I said, looking at her over my shoulder. She gave me a reassuring smile that didn't assure me.

"I'm not pregnant," she said staunchly.

"Okay, good. I believe you." I took her arm and curled mine inside hers. We were linked by our elbows.

"But if I were..."

"What?"

"I don't think I'd know who the father is."

"Oh my God, you are so white trash."

"I know," she said laughing. I was laughing too. We walked down the hall towards Dakota's apartment trying to keep our laughter from echoing in the hallway. The plush carpet did a good job of muffling our voices.

Just before we reached her door, Dakota whispered in my ear, "Not a word about Panty Man." As if I'd say anything. If she only knew how I preferred to avoid that subject. I gave her a look. In return she put her finger over her lips. When we got to her doorway, we quickly straightened ourselves out. I took my arm from hers, opened both doors and walked into the marble foyer. I always use both doors so I can make a grand entrance. Sitting beside the Mother Theresa that lives in all of us, is a very ostentatious Scarlet O'Hara. Dakota insists I am the only one who does this. I know for a fact that Kal does it too. He claims he has to open both doors to get his hockey bag through the entrance. Yeah, right.

A full-length mirror faced me. I couldn't see my entire figure because a huge table stood in front of the mirror, and on top of the table was a vase filled with an oversized bouquet. The flowers were pretty, but did there have to be quite so many? I turned to see my profile.

"Gorgeous dress," Dakota said, closing the double doors.

"Don't you just love it?"

"Yes, where did you get it?"

"Oh, I found this great store at the mall."

"Really?"

"Yes," I said kicking off my shoes, and moving onto the hardwood flooring. Kal was in the living room sprawled on the couch. His skin was a glorious bronze, while his hair had been sun bleached an off-white color.

"Where's your surf board?" I asked him. He didn't have his shirt on, but when you look that good, aren't clothes kind of sinful?

"Hi Sharon," he said lifting himself off the couch like Olympian Mitch Gaylord. I offered my cheek and he gave me the perfunctory kiss. I could smell his cologne and it made something in the pit of my stomach stir. I had to remind myself that I don't find blonds attractive. Not even one with a body that could give Mr. Universe a run for his money.

"What have you been doing all summer? You look like a beach bum." Why did I say bum?

"Oh, I had a job as a roofer for a while."

"Wow," I said flopping down on the couch. "You can do stuff like that?"

"He got fired," Dakota piped in. She reached for my wine.

"This is not for you," I said hanging onto it.

"Who is it for then?" She put her hands on her hips and waited.

"Me," I said selfishly. "I've had a rotten night and I'm here to drink."

"What's the matter?" Kal asked, taking a seat beside me. He looked so sweet. I could've put my head on his shoulders and confessed everything. He had really round deltoids. Round and brown. Mmm, yummy.

"Kal, can you..." Dakota made a motion with her hands for him to beat it.

"Sure, sure, no probs." Kal got up and went into the bedroom. He's not allowed in Dakota's office. It had become a lady's only room since we joined Ashley Madison.

Dakota rolled her eyes, after him.

"We can't talk here."

"Do you want to go out on the terrace?" I asked pushing myself off the couch. I'm not really the outdoors type, however on an evening like this, when the sky is dotted with thousands of stars and the temperature is mild, I can make an exception. It was a perfect night to be out with a lover.

"What were you and Kal doing before I arrived?" I asked, worried that I might have interrupted the start of something sexual between them.

"Nothing. Why?"

"Because I feel like I've intruded."

"I was reading," Dakota made some typing motions with her fingers. I nodded. She'd been online. "Kal's been watching TV." Dakota pretended to be sleeping with her mouth open. I started to laugh. She sat down beside me, and whispered in my ear, "He's such a lazy fuck."

"What does he do now that he's not a roofer?" I whispered back.

"What he did before his stint as a roofer; sweet fuck all."

"Have you seen his abs? I bet he does five hundred sit-ups a day."

"News flash, honey, sit ups can't pay the mortgage."

"Pity," I said.

"Humph," Dakota sighed and slouched into the down pillows on the couch.

"Do you want me to leave?" I asked, sliding sideways on the couch so I could recline.

"No, of course not, silly. Come on, we're going out. You look too pretty to sit around here." Dakota grabbed my wrist and pulled me out of my reclining position.

"Put your wine in the fridge. I'm going to get ready." I went into the kitchen. There were plastic containers of Chinese food on the stainless steel countertop. I didn't realize how hungry I was until I caught sight of the fried rice, garlic spare ribs, and almond *guy ding*. I put my wine in the wine fridge beneath the counter.

"Can I have your leftovers?" I hollered. There was no answer. I took that as a yes. I grabbed a plate from the cupboard and started to fill it.

"Sharon?" I jumped six feet.

"What?" I snapped.

"Don't eat that."

"I'm starving," I said, continuing to load my plate. "I haven't had any supper."

"If you eat that shit, it'll be your last supper."

"What's wrong with it?" I said taking a bite off the top of an egg roll.

"Well for starters, it's been there for three days."

"Three days?" I yelped, spitting out the egg roll into the napkin Dakota offered.

"Yup," she said pitching the napkin into the garbage bin.

"Why?"

"Kal ordered it for his lunch, or whatever, and it's been there ever since."

"Shouldn't he throw it out, or put it in the fridge, or something?"

"He's waiting for me to do it, and you know what, I'm tired of cooking and cleaning. Do I look like fucking Betty Crocker?" I took that as a rhetorical question and didn't answer.

"Let's get out of here," I said dumping the contents of the plate into the garbage bin. I put the plate in the dishwasher and rinsed my hands.

"Why can't he be like you?" Dakota asked whimsically.

"Because guys like him can't be housebroken."

Dakota and I left her condo and walked south, then west. We were both silent, except for the occasional noises from my tummy. We'd been walking for about ten minutes when Dakota finally spoke.

"I dumped Panty Man." Well wasn't that the best news I'd heard all day. I hoped the schmuck was heartbroken.

"I knew there was something eating you," I said, maintaining an even tone.

"It wasn't a matter of something eating me, it was more a case of someone *not* eating me that was the problem." We both giggled.

"If it's any consolation, I haven't had sex in seven months."

"Seven months?"

"Seven months, three days, fourteen hours, and fifty two minutes," I made up the last three stats, but they weren't that far off, and the seven months, sadly, was absolutely true. Dakota laughed hysterically. She grabbed me.

"Stop laughing," I said pushing her off my arm. "It's not that funny." Dakota continued to laugh.

"It's not just your horrible life, it's the irony of our lives. Oh Sharon, you're the best. You always make me feel so good."

"Yes, I think I was a court jester in a previous life," I theorized.

"Maybe, or maybe you were like one of those really wise women."

"If I was, I lost all my wisdom during the whole death and rebirth trauma."

"Oh no, you haven't. You're wise beyond your years."

"Tell that to Dogbiscuit. He thinks I'm a foolish spendthrift."

"Just ignore Scrooge. I have a feeling you're going to forget all about him soon."

"Unfortunately, every time I roll over in bed, I'm reminded of him."

"That's because you should be in bed with someone else."

"Tell me about it."

"Did you have a date tonight?"

"Yes," I said, smiling, even though my meeting with Steve didn't have a happy ending. Dakota and I continued walking until we found a small bistro. Along the way, I told her all about my night. By the time we were seated and had agreed to forgo dinner for dessert, my entire story had been told, including the search for the Muscat.

"Well," Dakota said, putting her menu down, "the first thing you have to do is start on your next lead."

"Did you decide what you're having?"

"Yes, the double chocolate mud cake."

"That's what I was going to have."

"Take the cheese cake," Dakota's confident tone sounded more like a strict order. I'd had enough of that for one night.

"Okay, Skeletor," I said, looking over my shoulder like I thought he might be around.

"Sorry," Dakota said, grinning. She didn't look sorry.

The waiter must have noticed that Dakota's menu was closed because he came over. "Ready to order?"

"Are you ready?" Dakota asked me.

"I'll have the cheesecake and an Earl Grey tea," I said, surrendering my menu before I could change my mind.

"I'll also have an Earl Grey tea, but I want the chocolate mud cake." Dakota practically flung her menu at the waiter. I felt sorry for him. He was expecting some kind of acknowledgment, but Dakota rarely flirts with those who serve her. She thinks it's vulgar.

"Okay, so who have you been sending messages to?" she asked me.

"No one special."

"You have been corresponding with a few men, though, right? Not just, what do you call him, Skeletor?"

"Yes, but I don't think there's anyone as good as Skeletor."

"Skeletor wasn't good, remember? He turned out to be a card-carrying, nature-obsessed, tofu-eating, tree-hugging, militaristic, vegetarian freak."

"Oh, right,." I said. "Thanks for the reminder. I don't want to forget those virtues."

"You're welcome. Now, what's wrong with the guys you're corresponding with?"

"Nothing's wrong with them, but nothing is right either."

"Okay, who's the hottest?"

"Mr. Bombastic."

"That's a fantastic name. Meet him tomorrow."

"I can't," I said in a whiny tone.

"Then meet him next week." I made a face. "What? What's his problem?"

"I dunno. He seems weird or shy or something. His messages are always so brief."

"I'd take that as a sign he's a busy man. He's probably very straightforward."

"I wouldn't know. His messages don't really reveal anything except that he's interested in meeting me."

"What more do you want?"

"Skeletor asked me philosophical stuff that got me thinking."

"Well, he turned out to be a nut. So, next!"

"Mr. Bombastic seems kind of disinterested. He's not really pursuing me aggressively."

"Mr. Bombastic can't be any worse than Elephant Man, Dinky, or Skeletor."

"We don't know that for certain."

"I'll bet on it."

"Okay, I'll meet him," I said, thinking I could arrange a coffee date that could be over in an hour.

"If he turns out to be a dud, I'll take you to Paris the next weekend I'm off," Dakota promised.

"What happens if he turns out to be some kind of wonderful?"

"Then you win. You'll have found what you've been looking for."

"I still want to go to Paris."

"You won't want to go without him. Trust me, when men are good, they are very, very good."

"But when they're bad, they're worse than Dogbiscuit."

Mr. Bombastic's style changed the moment I sent the five-word message, which read: *I want to meet you*. Almost immediately, he sent back a note requesting a lunch date at the Prince Hotel. I was reluctant to agree, because I wasn't feeling any kind of vibe between us. I just wanted a fast meeting, so I could tell Dakota he was a loser and collect my round-trip ticket to Paris. I sent back a message asking him to meet me for coffee. I got another message, which said only: *When can I take you to lunch?*

I loved his I-won't-take-no-for-an-answer attitude. Since we were eating on his dime, I didn't have anything to lose except a few hours of work, and I certainly wasn't going to complain about that. I sent another message: *Thursday* is all it said. He sent back: *1:30 Prince Hotel*. Do you see what I mean about brief?

Once I had the date finalized, I had to face the daunting task of finding something to wear. I went into my bedroom closet and began searching for the perfect outfit. McKenzie came in just after I discovered a skirt I've never worn. The tags were still attached.

"Mommy, what are you doing?"

"Shopping," I said, looking through my shirts that still had tags attached. I don't know why I never got around to wearing some of these things.

"Why don't you go to a store?"

"Daddy says I spend too much money."

"Oh, do you?"

"I'm not sure. I'm going to take a break from stores though."

"All stores?"

"Yes, I think so."

"Even Toys 'R' Us?" Mackenzie's face was etched with worry.

"No, of course not honey. We still have to get toys for you and Conner." I smiled at her. She smiled back, obviously relieved.

"And something for Margaret," she shouted.

"Do you think Margaret wants toys?"

"She wants a boyfriend." Mackenzie put her chubby hands over her mouth and giggled.

"How do you know that?"

"She said so."

"Okay, we'll get her a boyfriend."

"Where do boyfriends come from?"

"From the Internet, but don't tell dad."

On Thursday morning, I got out of bed as soon as I heard Dogbiscuit leave. I had all the time in the world since I was going to call in sick. I had a bath and a leisurely breakfast. Margaret shot me some quizzical looks while I nibbled on my French toast. As soon as she left with the kids, I ran to my bedroom and called work. The supervisor of my department, Edward, is a really nice man. He's round with a ruddy complexion that always earns him the role of Santa at our annual Christmas parties. I told him I was feeling very sick.

"I think it might be stomach flu," I moaned.

"Really?" came Edward's concerned voice over the line. He's the sort of chap who'd never believe someone like me would call in sick to go on a date with a married man. I had a pretty good work record, despite Ralph's disparaging perspective on the matter.

"Yes, I can't keep anything down," I said, coughing because vomiting and diarrhea are too hard to convey over the phone. Hopefully the cough was enough evidence that I was ill.

"Well, we'll see you tomorrow then?"

"Probably," I said. I used to get caught on that one all the time, by answering with a definite yes. Now, I like to keep everyone guessing. It makes my illness seem more credible.

As soon as I hung up, I started on my hair and makeup. In the back of my closet, beside my designer duds, I found a cute little black and white dress. The dress was divided into eight large rectangular panels, four covered the front and four the back. The rectangles alternated between black and white, forming an enlarged version of a checkerboard. It had a real sixties mod look to it. I loved it, yet I'd never worn it. If Dogbiscuit took me out once in a while, I might have a reason to wear some of my nice clothing.

I swept my hair up in a high ponytail and slipped into my platform sandals. It was only noon. I was actually going to be early. I had to get out of the house before Margaret returned, because she'd would definitely want to know why I wasn't at work. I couldn't fool her with the sick routine, at least not in this dress.

I slipped out of my house like a cat burglar, looking first to the left, then to the right. I managed to get away without being spotted. I should have driven straight to the hotel, but I had an hour-and-a-half to spare. I needed stamps, so I went to the post office. It should have taken seven minutes max, but there was an impossible line. The longer I waited, the more I felt I had to see it through to the end. When I finally got to the desk, it was 12:45. I practically ran from the post office, stuffing my stamps into my purse. I shouldn't have bothered, because as I peeled out of the parking lot, I got stuck in lunchtime traffic. I really wanted to be on time for a change. When I arrived at the hotel, it was 1:35. I couldn't find a parking spot close to the doors, even after circling twice. I gave up and parked far away. I would have sprinted to the doors, but my sandals only allowed a shuffle, skip, half jog.

It was 1:43 when I finally got to the hotel's front door. There, leaning against the wall, was a gorgeous man. So gorgeous, in fact, that I gave him a double-take. He had dark hair, a tan almost as impressive as Kal's, and really piercing blue eyes. Regrettably, I had to dart past him.

"Sharon," the mellifluous voice stopped me in my tracks. I doubled back.

"Yes?"

"It's me, your one-thirty appointment."

"Oh my gosh. Hi," I said, extending my hand.

"How are you?"

"I'm late," I said moving closer to him. He was really handsome, even up close. The photographs I'd seen were all taken from a distance, so until I shook his hand, I only had a vague idea of what he'd look like. He looked much better than I'd imagined. He was very smartly dressed in his tailored sports coat and light blue shirt. His lack of tie made him look kind of rebellious.

"Don't worry about being late," he said. He grinned and I was almost struck blind by his dazzling white teeth.

"I'm really sorry. I'm not usually late," I said. Well, from now on I wouldn't be late,not with him waiting for me.

"You aren't? You look like the kind of gal who likes to keep men waiting."

"No, no, I'd never intentionally keep anyone waiting. Time is money." That was a Dogbiscuit quote. I wasn't sure if it was appropriate, but Mr. Bombastic laughed.

"What's your name?" I asked.

"Jared, but call me Jed."

"Okay," I smiled. He smiled back.

"Let's go," he said, leading me into the restaurant.

He was so divine, I had to pinch myself to make sure I wasn't dreaming. I wasn't dreaming. I was going to make him mine, mine, mine. All mine. This one was going to work out. I just knew it.

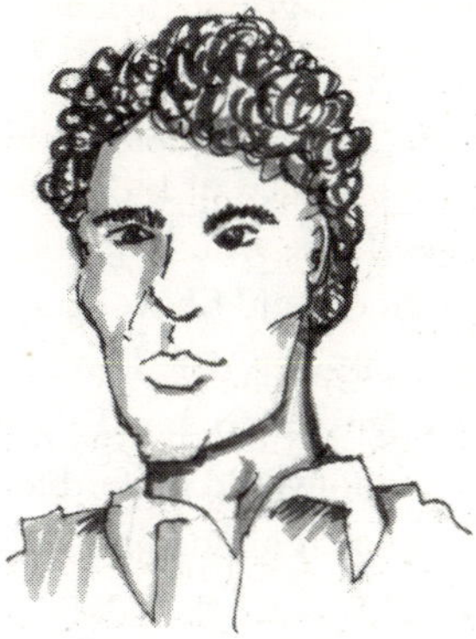

Chapter Eight:
Mr. Happily-Ever-After

That was the very best lunch I ever had. I can't remember what I ate, but I'm sure it was delicious. The restaurant adjacent to the Prince Hotel specializes in Japanese dishes. I ordered something with chicken and Jared ordered a huge platter of flesh-toned raw things. Normally, I would've found that rather revolting, but Jared used his chopsticks like a symphony conductor. He was so graceful, I couldn't take my eyes off him. I actually had to remind myself to eat. I can use chopsticks too, but I always look like I'm trying to knit a sweater with the food on my plate.

The best part of lunch was Jared. He was so fine. I can't believe I was so close to giving up. To think I almost let Skeletor, Elephant Man, and Dinky ruin my chances for sexual healing. I'm so glad I took Dakota's advice and tried yet another guy. It just goes to show, failure is the path of least persistence. My new mantra is going to be, "If at first you don't succeed, try, try again." My old rule of thumb was, "If at first you don't succeed, it's probably because of something

Dogbiscuit, said, or did, or something he forgot to do." If things don't work out with Jared—what am I saying, things will work out. They have to. He's just far too cute, and he knows how to dress himself like a man, instead of a midget auditioning for the part of an Umpa Lumpa in a *Willy Wonka* remake. I'm going to hang onto Jared with both hands, and my legs too, if necessary.

The only cloud on my silver lining was that I wasn't sure how Jared felt about me. When I looked at him, I thought some gorgeous blond should be hanging off his arm. A girl like Dakota, or Barbie. Jared looked a lot like the Sport and Shave Ken doll I received for my seventh birthday. I don't think Ken dated any of Barbie's dark-haired friends. When I subtly suggested to Jared during our lunch that he looked like the type of guy who would prefer blonds, he shook his head and said, "No, I don't think so." I almost jumped up out of my seat and cheered. Yes! Now all I had to do was convince him that I'm the sort of girl who can improve his life. Immeasurably. This was a huge task in itself, because, based on our looks alone, I am not sure we're even on the same page.

On a scale of one to ten, Jared was a perfect ten. Using the same beauty scale, I plateau around 8.275. This sort of thing shouldn't matter, especially since the most significant role I could ever have in his life is that of mistress, but it does. A man might stay married to a horse-faced woman, but no one would have an ugly woman as a mistress. Well, no one except Prince Charles. Come to think of it, President Clinton wasn't too selective either. Okay then, I guess looks don't matter all that much. Maybe it's true that a man is most attracted to what lies between the top of a woman's head and her shoulders. I always took that to mean the mouth, since most men spend countless hours fantasizing about receiving oral sex. However, the brain is located in the same vicinity. A great personality lasts a lot longer than a great face, as I'm sure Kathleen Turner will tell anyone with a box of donuts and a free hour.

It was a good thing Dogbiscuit was so fond of pointing out all my limitations and shortcomings. Everything he hated, was everything I'd try not to reveal to Jared. I promised myself I wouldn't talk too much about shopping. I wouldn't mention that my mother liked to go shopping with me. I wouldn't talk about all the money Dakota and I spent when we shopped together. I also wouldn't mention that I took an annual shopping trip to a new city every fall. Right, so what would we talk about? I'd have to cultivate an interest in something Jared liked. His wife had probably had to do that. I was very curious about the sort of woman who'd enthrall him enough to lead him down the aisle, but who lacked the cachet to keep him faithfully by her side.

While Jared and I were drinking the soup he'd ordered for our appetizer, I tried a few subtle openings for him to reveal something to me about his wife. He didn't take the bait. I tried again and received a monosyllable reply that told me nothing. I couldn't glean one tidbit of information about the woman. She could have been anybody, including a blond. Jared was an expert at avoiding subtle questions. I finally came out and asked, "What's your wife like?"

"Why? Are you interested in a threesome?"

"Are you?" I asked coyly.

"No, if you two hit it off, I might get jealous." I had to laugh.

"If she likes shopping, martinis, and sex, we're made for each other."

"She hates shopping, she'll go for the martini, but on the matter of sex, she's rather stoic."

"Stoic?" I repeated in a puzzled tone, not quite comprehending.

"Yes. You can sum up her love-making as the close-your-eyes-and-think-of-England method."

"Having your eyes open is the best part."

"Tell me about it," he said, sounding like he wanted details. He put his soupspoon down and focused on me.

"Do you prefer the lights on or off?" I asked.

"I not only keep the lights off, I also keep my eyes tightly shut, and if I had a blindfold I'd wear that too."

"Why?" I asked, intrigued by the image of him blindfolded.

"I can't stand her grin-and-bear-it face."

"Oh," I said nodding in sympathy. "How often do you put her through it?"

"I haven't touched her in three years."

"Three years? Oh my, you poor man." Even though I'd just met Jared, I felt it might be a gesture of goodwill to offer myself to him, strictly on humanitarian grounds, of course.

Jared finished his soup and pushed his bowl aside. He had long, elegant fingers and a big, fat, gold wedding ring. Was it really necessary for that ring to be so thick? I've seen shackles that were thinner.

"I haven't touched her in three years. But she's not the only cookie in the jar, is she?" Jared gave me a licentious grin that made my stomach flip-flop.

"That's right," I said quickly. I turned my attention to my soup. I was starting to feel hot all over, and I wasn't sure what was responsible for my sudden rise in temperature. Was it the spicy soup? Or was it the thought of Jared's long fingers caressing my bare skin?

"Pardon me?" I said. He was talking and I hadn't heard a word. Jared cleared his throat before speaking again. He raised his voice a tiny bit above the hushed tone he'd been using.

"I've had a couple of long-term relationships. Now I'm looking for something less stifling."

"Do you just want to play the field?"

"No, I want one woman. I'm a married man; I don't have the inclination to be seen with a different woman every time I straighten my tie."

"After all you aren't Hugh Hefner."

"That's right," he smiled. His teeth were so radiant, it made me smile too.

"Did the women you had affairs with want a lot of your time?"

"Sure. They were single. It was a mistake on my part to think I could satisfy them with the few hours I can spare."

How few? I wondered. I too could find myself in a similar predicament, wanting more of Jared's time than he could spare. An hour a week wasn't going to cut it with me either. I wanted to ask him how much time he had, but I didn't want him to think that becoming my lover would be a full-time job. Anyway, it would be rather presumptuous to assume he had any interest in me beyond lunch.

I drank some more soup, then I asked, "After a while, did the girls become too demanding?"

"Not the first one. With her it was more a problem of having incompatible goals. She was looking for a husband. I already had a wife. When I couldn't always be with her, she threw in the towel."

"And the second one?"

"The second girl was a brief affair. I was on the rebound."

"From the first girl?"

"Yeah, I was sort of fucked-up after the first one left. I'd had this idea that she'd always be there. I was greedy. I thought I could have her and my family. All the while, she was expecting me to leave my wife. Things came to a head a year ago during the Christmas holidays. She was alone and wanted me to be with her, but I wasn't prepared to leave my family. She delivered an ultimatum that I couldn't possibly meet, so we ended it. It was a difficult break and I should have kept to myself for a while, but I needed someone to help me forget. Do you know what I mean?"

"Yes," I said. I knew what he meant, even though I have never been in love with anyone other than Dogbiscuit, if you could call it that, and I've never suffered through a break-up. I knew because, in some ways, I was looking for the same thing; someone who could help me escape the pain of my life. I needed someone who would validate me as a woman and help me forget that I didn't love my husband, and that he probably didn't love me.

"You didn't love the second girl?" I asked.

"Not only did I not love her, I knew from the moment I met her that she was trouble."

"But you had a relationship with her anyway."

"Hindsight is twenty:twenty." Jared took a sip of water.

I took my soup spoon out of the bowl, and placed the bowl to the left side of the table. I looked at Jared and he was staring at me.

To break the silence, I asked, "How did you break up?"

"When she became a parasite, I had to shake her. First it was round the clock phone calls, then the constant whining about us spending more time together. There are only so many hours in a day. I was seeing her as much as my schedule would allowed. Some weeks, I saw her more often than I saw my wife."

As soon as Jared closed his mouth over the word wife, the waitress appeared in her blue and white kimono. Her face was a mask of indifference, but I was sure she knew Jared and I were having a clandestine luncheon. I could feel my face heating up with embarrassment. She deftly placed the food on the table and retreated with a slight bow. As soon as she'd left, Jared noticed my discomfort.

"What's the matter?"

"Nothing," I said, picking up my chopsticks.

"Are you uncomfortable being with me?"

"No," I said emphatically. How could he think that?

"Don't feel embarrassed. Do you think we're the first two people to have a rendezvous in a restaurant?"

"No, but..."

"People like us are the bread and butter of the hotel trade." He laughed. I laughed too.

"A lot of these places would go under if it weren't for us. They need us, we don't need them, so keep your chin up."

"Okay," I said. Jared unwrapped his chopsticks and began eating. I did the same. I concentrated on imitating Jared's skillful movements.

"What did you actually say in your break-up speech?" I don't know why I wanted all the details, but I did.

"I told her it was over."

"Did you take her to dinner first?"

"No. Is that how you handle your break-ups?"

"I've never had a break-up."

"Before you were married?'"

"Not ever."

"Really?" Jared asked, truly amazed. I nodded. He stared at me dumbfounded.

"Back to you," I said.

"She wouldn't leave me alone."

"She stalked you?"

"She stalked me day and night."

"Did you have to go to the police?"

"And risk having my wife find out? Not a chance. I dealt with her myself."

"What did you do?"

"I laid it on the line. I told her it was over, and I wanted her out of my life, permanently." He said this in the same gravelly voice contract killers use. If he meant to scare me, it worked. Even though we were still in the first stage of our potential relationship, I made a mental note not to engage in any stalking sprees should things become acrimonious.

"Don't give me that look." He sounded annoyed.

"What look?" Fear has a way of lighting up my face.

"Listen," he said leaning over the table, "I have a nine-year-old boy whom I love. I want him to have a mom and a dad. If anything gets in the way of that," he snapped his chopstick in half.

"Point taken," I said, shuffling uncomfortably on my chair. Where did I see those emergency exits?

"How about you?" Jared asked. He resumed eating with his broken chopstick.

"I don't have any stalkers, but at this point, I'd love one."

"No, you wouldn't," he said laughing.

"I think I would. A stalker is just a person with a lot of time on their hands who's totally crazy about you. What could be more flattering?"

"More flattering would be a person who truly cares about you and allows you the space and privacy you need to live your life the way you want to." After Jared said that, I relaxed again. That was a reasonable expectation only a really grounded person could articulate so well. A Mafioso-type would have had an entirely different perspective.

"Well, that's flattering, but at this sexless point in my life I'd welcome any man who--"

"Bullshit," he said, stopping me from saying anything more. I had to rethink my sentence.

"Okay, not any man." Not Dinky, nor Elephant Man, nor Skeletor.

"You want Prince Charming." For a moment I didn't say anything, because Dakota always says that to me. I had no idea my desires were so transparent.

"I want, something great because I don't have that now, and I never have. I know a lot of women marry the wrong person, but usually those women have wonderful memories of the guy they left behind. I don't. When things between my husband and I soured, I didn't have any sweet memories to console me."

"I know," he said.

"How do you know?"

"I can see it in your face and read it in your cryptic messages, and I can feel it now." Oh my God, I am so in love with this man.

"What cryptic messages?" I said, getting to the one thing he'd said that I didn't like.

"Every message from you was so loaded with double meanings and coded passages. I spent most of my time trying to read between the lines."

"That's funny because when I'm on Ashley Madison, I spend most of my time trying to read between the lies." Jared lifted his chin and laughed. He had a nice laugh, cheerful and infectious. I looked at his exposed neck and thought how wonderful it would be to sprinkle a trail of warm kisses along his throat.

"I was never sure you wanted anything more than to match wits with me."

"I thought you were totally disinterested in me."

"How could you think that? I kept writing to you, didn't I?"

Jared put his chopsticks down and looked me straight in the eyes. I met his gaze for as long as I could, then looked away. There was a really intense feeling building between us, and it made my heart thump in my chest, and my breath catch in my throat.

"I couldn't write much," he continued, "because half the time, I wasn't sure what to say."

"Well the last few messages were good."

"I'm glad I was finally able to please you." I loved the way he said "please you". I had a few more ideas of how he could please me, but I'd save those for later.

"Do you want my chopstick?" I said, offering it to him. He took it, and threw the broken one over his shoulder. That made me laugh. He laughed with me. I picked up the fork the waitress had set beside my plate.

"Thanks," he said.

"No problem. I'm better with a fork."

"With those long fingers I bet your hands are good with just about anything."

"Just about." I said, grinning wickedly. Jared smiled back at me and actually blushed!

When the waitress came to clear the plates, she offered dessert. I wanted to say yes, just so I could spend more time with Jared, but spoke before I could, and said, "Nothing else, thanks." When the check had been paid, Jared helped me to my feet, and we walked from the restaurant side by side. We collided into each other a couple of times, my shoulder against his arm.

"Do you want to come with me to my car?"

"Sure," I said, looking up into his handsome face. In my head I was praying he wasn't going to bring me to his car for a bring-and-brag.

When we got to his silver Audi, he told me to close my eyes. I covered my face with my hands. I heard him open, then shut, one of the doors.

"Open," he said. I took my hands away from my face and opened my eyes. Jared had a beautifully wrapped box in his hands.

"Sweets, for my sweet," he said.

"Oh, thank you," I took the box from him. I thought I should kiss him or something, but his cheek was so far away, I wasn't sure I could reach it without gripping his wide chest, and clinging to his narrow waist, and maybe ripping his shirt and jacket from his body.

"You're very welcome. Let me know how you enjoy them."

"I will. Why didn't you bring this into the restaurant?" I asked, lifting the box slightly. It was heavy.

"It would've been too much of a fuss."

"Sure, I bet you would've given these to your wife if you didn't like me," I teased him. He was a good sport and laughed.

"Shall I drive you to your car?" he said, opening the passenger door.

"No, that's okay." I couldn't trust myself in the confines of his slick automobile. Already, I was tempted to seduce him on the spot. The best thing to do was to play it safe and keep my distance. If I threw myself on him on our very first date, he would have no reason to see me again. Unless he was interested in an encore performance, and I wasn't sure in my sex deprived state anyone would want an encore with me.

"I had a wonderful time with you," he said.

"The pleasure was mine," I said clutching my hefty present. We shook hands, awkwardly even though I tried to convey telepathically, my desire for a kiss. Jared got into his car. I leaned against the driver's door.

"Are you sure I can't bring you to your car? I promise to keep my hands where you can see them." He grinned at me. Okay, so he was picking up some of my thoughts. Either that or his mind was also occupied with licentious thoughts.

"The problem is," I said seductively, "I would like to see your hands in all sorts of places where they probably shouldn't be."

"I won't tell if you don't."

"I think we better leave things as they are right now, so there is nothing to tell," I said, not meaning one word of what came out of my mouth.

"Okay, will you take a lift to your car?"

"Well," I said looking around the parking lot, "I'm not sure where I left it."

"I can help you find it," he offered gallantly. He patted the black leather passenger seat.

"I've got a remote starter," I said.

"Damn technology, it's making men obsolete."

"Not a chance," I said.

"Is there a use for me?" he asked leaning out of his car.

"I can think of plenty of uses for you," I said.

"We'll have to explore those."

"Call me and we can discuss it."

"I will," he said. You'd better, I thought to myself.

"Bye, Sharon," he said, starting his car.

"Ciao, Jared." I stood and watched him drive away. When he rounded the corner of parking lot and headed toward the exit, I got my feet to move in the direction of where I thought my car was parked. I spotted it in the far corner, nestled between a Cadillac and a Pathfinder. I walked to my car with a huge grin on my face.

I stayed happy all through Friday evening. I even smiled when Dogbiscuit asked, "Whose box of goodies?"

"Mine," I told him, moving the box away from his prying hands.

"What's inside?"

"Chocolates, cookies, coffee, tea, and biscuits."

"A bloody royal feast. I guess now that your closet is overstuffed with clothes you're going to want to start on the pantry."

"I didn't buy this. It was a gift."

"From whom?" Dogbiscuit's voice dripped with doubt and scorn.

"My lover," I said, fondling the package. Dogbiscuit burst out laughing.

"Right, Sharon, you have a lover. The battery operated kind I presume."

"Yes, that's right. And unlike you, he's able to satisfy me, because he just keeps going and going and going."

On Saturday, I checked my Ashley Madison mailbox and there was nothing from Jared. The voice mail for my cell phone was also devoid of any messages from him. My happy mood didn't feel so happy anymore. There was a message from my cousin Kate. She was wondering how I was making out with whatever I was up to. I hadn't talked to her since Mike had blown me off and I'd called her for advice. I made a mental note to call her later.

I oscillated between intense feelings of euphoria every time I ate something from my gift box, and deep feelings of depression every time I checked my voice mail. When I thought about the ninety-seven minutes (yes I'd calculated it!) I'd spent with Jared, I felt warm and tingly all over. I'm sure he had a good time, so why, oh why, hadn't he called me? I logged onto Ashley Madison and checked for messages. While I was on, I got an instant message from a guy who asked what I was looking for. I told him I wasn't looking for anyone anymore. I'd already found what I wanted. The guy sent back a message that said good luck, but I could sense a bit of hostility behind it. Why are some people resentful of other people's success?

Not that I was feeling very successful. There were five new messages in my mailbox, but none from Jared. I knew I should've answered at least one of them to stay in the game until I find my anti-Dogbiscuit, but I was feeling so blue, I logged off without reading any of them.

By Sunday I still hadn't heard from Jared. I checked my Ashley Madison mailbox. I had one new message from a guy called Romeo. As a rule, I avoid men who lack originality and creativity. I also can't stand guys with really crass nicknames like LickYourPussy and CumWithMe. Of course I'm not opposed to the activities, per se, in fact I respect a man who has a thorough knowledge of what a woman wants in bed—I just don't think he should use it as a name. I shudder to think what might appear online if we all started naming ourselves after our sexual preferences and activities.

Romeo had also sent me a message on Saturday, which I hadn't bothered to read, so I read it. I figured if it showed any promise, I'd read Sunday's message. It said he liked my profile very much and would love the chance to wine, dine and pamper me. Yes, he said pamper. That must be the latest online buzzword to woo women into the loser's den.

Romeo's Sunday message asked me to respond even if it was to say get lost. I was tempted to send back a message that said: *Get lost.* I looked up Romeo's profile first. He was forty-two, which meant he was probably closer to fifty. He was over six feet tall and he described himself as fit. His photo was a close-up of his face, which was pleasing and friendly in a guy-next-door way. I didn't like the fact that he had no shot of his body. That left too much to chance, like he might be a tub of lard with a lean face. There are people like that. They're the ones you make eye contact with at red lights, because they look good and so do their cars. But if you pull over, and encourage them to do the same, you might be very disappointed, as Dakota and I once found out.

We were on our way back from a cocktail lounge early last March. We'd gone out that night to see a jazz singer who was so adept at singing the blues, both Dakota and I were ready to kill ourselves after the first set. We saved each other by leaving. Then we stopped at the Dairy Queen for two large Pecan Parfaits. That cheered us up. When we pulled out of the parking lot, we made a sharp right and hit a red light. Dakota noticed the car next to us, a silver Mustang. The driver had a cute face. He looked like a very young Kevin Costner. I wasn't that interested because, you know, I'm so not into blonds. Dakota was bouncing up and down on the seat, and that got the guy to look at us. She hit a button and the window of her Mercedes coupe, slid down.

"Hey," she said, waving like she was the Homecoming Queen.

"Hi girls," the guy called back.

"Pull over," Dakota said.

"Ay, ay, captain." The guy gave a salute. He wasn't smiling, he looked scared.

"Dakota," I said," I think that guy thinks we're undercover cops."

"No, he doesn't," she said, laughing. "This isn't an Intrepid."

The light turned green and the mustang signaled and carefully entered our lane. We followed it through the intersection. The Mustang pulled over to the right, and we did the same. Dakota shut off the ignition and sprang out like it was the General Lee and she was Daisy Duke. I got out reluctantly. Dakota went over to the driver's side of the Mustang, and I went to the front passenger window. The driver opened both windows, but he didn't get out.

"Hey dude," Dakota said.

"Hi, how are you?" the guy answered back.

Both Dakota and I stuck our heads through the open windows of the guy's car.

"What's your name, fella'?" I asked. Why did I suddenly sound like Daisy Duke?

"Tom," he said. He was looking at me and I was looking at his thighs. You know how when you sit down your thighs spread out and look twice as fat as normal? Well Tom's legs were so fat, they looked like they'd morphed together. There was just one huge lap on the car seat, and it was spilling over the gearbox and grazing the passenger door. Tom couldn't even say "Get in" because we would've had to ask "Where?" He didn't get out of his car because he probably couldn't lift himself without an ass paddle.

"Do you know how fast you were traveling, Tom?" that came from Dakota.

"I wasn't traveling, I was stopped at a red light," Tom spoke to Dakota and then gave me a sycophantic smile. I looked over Tom's head at Dakota. I lifted my chin slightly. I pulled my head out of Tom's car and leaned over the car roof. Dakota got my message and lifted her head. I puffed my cheeks out like a chipmunk and pursed my lips. Dakota started laughing.

"Hey," yelled Tom.

I bent my head back into the passenger window.

"What's up buddy?"

"Are you guys cops or chicks?"

"We're cop-loving chicks," Dakota said

"I'm not a cop either, but I could show you some love."

"Give me your number," Dakota said.

As I started walking back to Dakota's car, I heard Tom ask, "Do you girls want to do a three-way?" I was tempted to tell him AT&T does three-ways. Instead, I just kept on walking till I reached the car. I let myself in and slumped in the leather seating.

When Dakota finally got back to the car, she burst out laughing, before she had the door closed.

"Oh, my God," she said laughing, "what a total disappointment."

"He suckered you," I said, giving her a sidelong glance.

"Who would put such a gorgeous head on Fat Albert's body?"

"I dunno, but some people were wondering the same thing about Delta Burke and Kirstie Ally."

"Did you see his legs?" Dakota asked as she wiped tears from her eyes.

"His knees were bigger than my head," I said. That sent Dakota off into another fit of mad laughter. Ahead of us, Tom's car started to move. I watched Tom pull out from the curb and enter the flow of traffic. I wanted to toot the horn at him, but Dakota was bent over the steering wheel, laughing. I hope he isn't still expecting her to call. The little scrap of paper he wrote his number on was used as a wrapper for Dakota's chewed gum ages ago.

"I've never seen legs so big, have you?" Dakota put on her seat belt, and tried to get the key in the ignition, but couldn't because her arms were quivering from laughter. I considered her question. No, I didn't think I'd seen anyone with legs quite that large either. Although I didn't think Tom's biggest problem was the size of his legs. His figure flaw was that he had a close to normal upper body, while his legs were at least three times the size of an ordinary fat guy's. Usually you see that type of figure on women. Some people call it a pear-shaped figure. I call it fat. Well, not to their face.

"His legs looked like someone had stuck a hose up his pants and filled them with air," I said.

"He had a nice face though," Dakota offered, starting the car.

"Yup," I said. It was best not to argue.

Romeo's picture reminded me of Tom. Romeo was a brown-eyed blond. He had nicely arched brows over his eyes. Kal would've been jealous. I decided to send him a message. It wasn't like I had anything better to do.

Hey Romeo,

Thanks for writing (twice!). I'm very busy with all my suitors. It's tough being popular, but I'm still Sharon from the block. I think I can fit you in. If you're fit, fun, and energetic, I could be the Juliet of your dreams!

I could only hope he wouldn't miss the subtle point I was making about being fit and energetic, just as I hadn't missed his promise of wining, dining and pampering.

There was still no word from Jared. I searched through my old messages and found Jared's first. I clicked on it so I could re-read it.

Hello Sharon,

When I pamper a woman, I offer the very best there is, and when I offered it to you, I had nothing less in mind. If you're interested in experiencing unparalleled joys, I'm the man for you.

How could I have ignored that? Oh my God, I can't believe I didn't arrange a meeting with him immediately after reading that the first time. I guess I must have been really jived about Skeletor. Now I can't remember what was so great about him. I did like his philosophical ravings and those intellectual questions he attached to every message. Although, come to think of it, I don't think I ever responded to any of those questions correctly. Oh well.

That night, Mackenzie allowed me to read *Cinderella* for her bedtime story. It wasn't my favorite fairy tale, but I liked that the prince came looking for Cinderella. And of course, I loved the happily-ever-after ending. I lived for it. Someday my own Prince Charming was going to rescue me from my life with Dogbiscuit. I just wasn't sure when.

That Monday, I spent my morning hours with the kids. When Margaret left with them for the park, I got ready for work and arrived on time for a change. As soon as I arrived at the office, I got straight to it. No idling at the coffee machine. No small-talk with my office mates. I sat down and buried my head in my files. Around twelve-thirty my phone rang. I reached for my office phone before realizing it was my cell. My cell is usually off, but when I'm meeting someone, I like to have it on. I must have left it on since Friday. I hadn't used it since. Whenever I check for messages I use my landline, so my cell usually sits by my phone. That's the only way I can find it when I'm heading out. I pulled it out of my purse and checked the battery. It was at a mid-level.

"Hello," I said.

"Hello, Sharon, how are you?"

"Jared?" My heart did a flip-flop and landed in my throat.

"It's me doll. How was your weekend?"

"Fine," I said, not letting on that I'd been miserable for two days.

"I thought about you all weekend."

"Really?" I was trying so hard not to sound like a lovelorn high-school girl.

"Yes. I hated leaving you on Friday. You found your car okay?"

"Yes," I said. I wanted to hear more about him missing me.

"Are you free for lunch today?"

I wanted to say yes, but I couldn't leave the office. I'd just arrived.

"No, what about tomorrow?" I crossed my fingers.

"I'm out of town tomorrow," he said. Shit, I can't believe this is happening to me.

"What about Wednesday?" I said, holding my breath and crossing my fingers.

I thought I heard Jared flip a page. He must have been checking his Day Runner.

"That might work."

"Where should I meet you?" I uncrossed my fingers, took a breath and reached for a pen and my note pad.

"There're some good restaurants on King. Why don't we meet at the Holiday Inn?"

"Okay. In the lobby?" As opposed to the honeymoon suite.

"Yes, does one o'clock work for you?" he asked.

"Two o'clock is better." That way I could arrive at work early, and then leave for a doctor's appointment. Depending on when Jared and I finished lunch, I might even return to work. Might. There was a part of me that wanted to show Ralph I was capable of cultivating good work habits, conducting myself professionally, and maintaining an excellent attendance record. But there was also a part of me that enjoyed a slow-paced stroll through the downtown, looking at shop windows, and watching people eat, as they sat at the curbside patios. In a few weeks, we'll all be bundled up in coats. I didn't want to spend the last few days of summer locked away in an office cubicle.

"Fine, you're in my book," Jared said. I wondered what he'd written. *Sex with Sharon @ 2,* or *Lunch :) with Sharon @ 2:00pm.* It didn't really matter. The most important thing was that he'd called. The second most important thing was that he wanted to see me again. I had another date with Jared! Soon he was going to be mine. Mine, all mine.

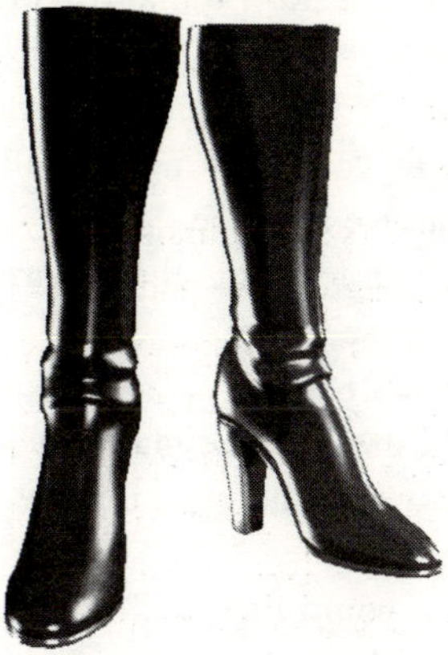

Chapter Nine:
Gold Fingers

Dogbiscuit was driving my nerves into the ground. I knew he wasn't deliberately trying to antagonize me, but just his presence made me want to run screaming from the room. We'd been rampaging through the house as though we were playing some insane game of musical chairs. I didn't know why he'd suddenly developed a prolonged interest in me. I was pretty much the same Sharon I always had been, just a little happier I suppose, and a little less crinkly around the edges.

The happiness I could attribute to Jared, and the reduced crinkles to a fantastic new moisturizer I'd discovered at the Body Shop. The night before, I'd been lying on the bed in the guest room, where I'd been spending a lot of my time since Dogbiscuit had given me the idea a few weeks back, when out of the blue, in he walked.

"Sharon I've been looking all over for you." he said coming close to the bed.

I thought he was going to unzip his pants and demand some action. I rolled over on my stomach, keeping my *Cosmo* open to the page on how to improve my orgasms.

"What is it?" I asked, keeping my face between the pages, although I'd lost my place on the page and my concentration.

"What have you been doing in here?" He sounded so lecherous.

"I've been cleaning," I said. I found my place and tried to block him out.

"Cleaning! Humph. Your cleaning bears a remarkably self-indulgent resemblance to your cooking." I rolled over on my back, keeping the magazine above my face.

"Look," I said, without lowering the magazine, "I'm very busy at the moment. Can you please leave?"

"I came in here to talk to you."

"What is it then?" I dropped the magazine on the bed and let out a heavy sigh so he'd know just how put out I was about having to talk to him.

"I was wondering if you'd like to..."

"No," I said firmly. I rolled off the bed and walked out from room. So that's why he'd been skulking after me like an *Enquirer* photographer trying to catch a big-money celebrity off guard.

"Sharon," he called after me. I ran down the stairs and went into the kitchen. He followed me.

"Can you please hear me out?" He ran past where I was standing and stood between me and the fridge. I crossed my arms over my chest.

"I'm not interested in sex," I told him. "I'm on a diet and sex is strictly prohibited, along with salt, soft drinks, and starchy foods."

"Sex!" he shouted, "I'm not talking about sex."

"You aren't?" I said, starting to feel foolish.

"No, I wanted to know if you'd come with me to the company picnic."

"So, you mean just now, upstairs, you weren't asking for sex?"

"Of course not," he said contemptuously, like I'd just offered him a roadkill and broccoli sandwich.

"Oh," I said. Why didn't he want to have sex? Was it normal for a man to go this long without any sexual activity? Even I had surpassed my previous best, which was set during the six-month waiting period between my first sexual experience with Dogbiscuit and the second. Now into my eighth month without sex, not only was the record shattered, I was about to set a new one.

"Will you come?" Dogbiscuit was pleading with me to attend his picnic.

"I have to think about it," I told him, feeling more and more angry that his trailing me around wasn't due to horniness.

"Say yes, Shar. You know you want to," he cajoled. Did he really think I was some idiot who didn't know he only wanted me come so I could look after the kids, while he networked with his drunken colleagues?

"What's in it for me?" I asked, like a true mercenary.

"Sex, if you want it," he said. He shook his hips like he was attempting to make a hula-hoop spin. Because he's so thin and unbelievably awkward, he looked a bit like he was suffering from cerebral palsy. I thought it was rather pathetic that he was offering sex as a reward. He didn't seem to realize that sex is like football. The more you do it, the better you get at it, and the more you want to do it. At least every Monday night anyway, which would have been a vast improvement in our case. My cousin Kate has sex every day. Every day! Poor Dogbiscuit had no idea that sexual intimacy could be so much more than a matrimonial duty. Was there any better pastime than sex with someone you love, or, if not that, with someone you didn't hate intensely?

"I'll take sex," I told him flatly, "but not with you." My few brief moments making out with Dinky had taught me that there was kissing, and then there was the wet slobbering, mouth wrestling Dogbiscuit tried to pass off as competent passion. Sucker fish show more finesse sucking the algae from the sides of fish tanks. I can still remember my first kiss with Dogbiscuit.

We were sitting in the park and he asked, "Can I kiss you?"

I was so surprised all I could think to say was, "Why do you want to do that?"

His response had been immediate."Because I like you."

I dipped my head to avoid his stringy lips, and said, "I don't think we should." I wasn't sure I wanted Dogbiscuit to be the first guy I ever kissed. Even then, he seemed inadequate and wrong for me.

"I want you to be my girlfriend," he said. When I heard that, I was immediately overcome with a sense of gratitude. At last, I was to be someone's girlfriend. So what if that someone looked like Mr. Bean?

"Okay," I said, surrendering to the promise of finally being someone's girlfriend. That first kiss I shared with Dogbiscuit was dry from my end, and gushy wet from his. My mouth was shut tightly against his probing tongue, which pushed against my teeth like a log caught in a dam. My teeth were clenched so tightly, I gave myself a headache. That kiss wasn't memorable in the way a first kiss should be. In fact, it only remained in my memory because it was so very different from what my young mind had imagined.

I'd cut my teeth on romance novels. Really. When I was a young toddler with legs so fat they couldn't be trusted to stand, let alone walk, I'd hoist myself to a standing position, using any available furniture. One day I pulled myself up on a bookshelf, and it tipped over. Down came a rain of paperback novels about lonely nurses, and secretaries. Misses in search of their Misters. I escaped unharmed, but there was a little corner of my left front tooth missing when my mother picked me up and brushed me off. She said the odd thing was, that although I was shaken up, I didn't cry. Not even from fright. So maybe I came to my love of romance novels from my near-death experience. I don't know. All I know is, when all the other grade four girls were reading *Charlotte's Web* and *Little House on the Prairie*, I was reading Harlequin romance novels. With the exception of Judy Bloom, and a few others like her, the women writing fiction for kids just didn't put enough excitement between the covers to keep me turning pages. I waited forever for Nancy Drew to get her groove on with one of the Hardy Boys.

Reading all those romance novels helped me become one of the best readers in the class. I could decode words like nobody's business. The downside was that I walked away from those books with a very unrealistic picture of life. As a direct result of filling my head with so many Harlequins and Silhouettes, I actually came to believe in modern-day fairy tales. I was convinced that one day I'd meet a dashing businessman who seemed like a regular working guy, but in reality, he'd be a multi-millionaire with a castle and a sports car. When he kissed me, my breath would catch in my throat and I'd swoon from the pleasure of the contact of his lips against my soft, pliant mouth.

What actually happened was my breath was knocked out by Dogbiscuit's mild, but ever-present, halitosis. It would have induced a faint, but the sensation of someone's spittle drying on my lips was so revolting, it heightened all my senses and I stayed uncomfortably alert. The memory of Dogbiscuit's saliva drying on my lips, stayed with me for a long time. Too long. It made me wonder about a sentence I'd once read in one of those triple-X romance novels with the red covers. Speaking to herself, the heroine said, "I can still feel his kiss on my lips." She made it seem like a pleasant thing, but let me clarify for those who have been fortunate enough not to know what this means. For the record, feeling someone's kiss on your lips long after the kiss has ended is, in a word, disgusting.

Was her lover the same kind of slobbering buffoon I got saddled with? Not only is Dogbiscuit a terrible, terrible, kisser, he's also absolutely and completely dismal when it comes to any sexual activities. I don't know how adept he is at masturbation, but I suspect that if you talked to his penis, it would have a few complaints about what his hand was doing.

Dogbiscuit's main problem is that he has no real interest in sexual gratification. Therefore, he doesn't know how, or even why, he has to please his partner. That would be the long-suffering me. He isn't actually too bad at the in and out, in and out, part. However, if he's required to do anything else, he does it so poorly, you'd think he was acting out of spiteful discontent. In particular, his oral is so bad that just the thought of it sets my teeth on edge.

Back in the day when my only sexual outlet was Dogbiscuit, I had to suffer through it, hoping he'd come to the realization that "eat me" is not a literal term. Chewing has no part in cunnilingus. For the health and happiness of the recipient, anything involving teeth and grinding should be avoided.

Before my hotel assignation with Dinky, I didn't have a real appreciation of Dogbiscuit's lack of amorous skill. Now that I knew about the potential delights, I simply couldn't go back. I could never again settle for Dogbiscuit's two tweaks followed by six thrusts and a shudder.

"Why don't you want me? You think you can do better than me?" he asked. I pushed him aside and grabbed a Fresca from the fridge.

"No, I don't. I think you're the very best thing I can have. That's why I married you."

"Don't waste your sarcasm on me." Gee, how did he know I was being sarcastic?

"I'm trying to have a real moment with you," I said, using my Dr. Phil voice.

"Well, what I really want to hear is yes, you will be coming to the picnic."

"Okay, yes," I said, growing tired of him.

"Thank you, Sharon. I would kiss you, but I know how you feel about my germs."

"Money speaks louder than words," I said heading out of the kitchen. I was going back upstairs to finish my article. I started my Kiegel exercises on my way up the stairs. That's the first step to increasing my orgasmic power.

I heard Dogbiscuit call out, "Sharon, you're my wife, not an escort."

"Please don't remind me. I'm trying to wean myself off Zanax." I wasn't really on the drug, but I thought I'd throw that out just to irritate Dogbiscuit. I was feeling very good at that moment. I thought the picnic might even be fun, but I'd be damned if I was going to let him know. Why should I agree without some sort of compensation? "An eye for an eye", that's the basic code of marriage. Or is it, "You wash my back, I'll wash yours"?

To say I was frustrated beyond measure by the loveless, sexless void that had become my life, is to state the obvious. I kept dreaming about sex. Each morning I'd wake up to this bizarre feeling that the night before, Dogbiscuit and I had actually engaged in foreplay or some mild sexual activity. Usually my dreams would end before penetration became an issue.

The other day, for example, I fell asleep in the living room and dreamt that Dogbiscuit came in, pulled my panties off and started to go down on me. As I was dreaming, I realized the entire experience was a dream because, instead of withering on the chair in agony, I actually found the experience pleasant, although, in the dream, I was really not feeling much of anything, which is, of course, preferable to Dogbiscuit's painful gnawing.

The mornings after my sex dreams were always a little disconcerting, because I was never one-hundred percent certain that it was a dream, or if it had actually occurred. Sometimes, I dreamed about having sex with other men. I dreamed about Jared. I really liked that dream. When I awoke, I had an intensely euphoric feeling, which crashed and burned the moment I realized Jared wasn't asleep beside me. I went back to bed, but I couldn't re-ignite the warm glow of contentment I'd had when I first opened my eyes, expecting to find Jared.

I also dreamt about doing it with Kal. That dream scared the shit out of me. I woke up drenched in sweat with my heart beating so loudly, I was sure Dogbiscuit was going to jump out of his slumber and make a grab for the sledgehammer. He keeps the hammer under the bed in order to protect us against any would-be burglars, should anyone make it past the security system, the motion sensitive stadium lights, and the sprinklers. Of late, Dogbiscuit had been watering the lawn in the dead of night. He was working on a theory. Personally, I thought he was in competition with the guy across the street. I wondered if either one of them realized there was no prize for the best lawn. In fact there was an anti-prize, since dogs seem to like to do their duty on the softest, greenest grass available. After all, you never see a dog taking a dump on front yards that look like clay infields, do you?

Anyway, back to me. I wanted to discuss my recent dreams with Dakota, but I couldn't. She might have found the thought of Kal and me getting freaky between the sheets objectionable. Even though she said she wanted to dump him, I was sure that, not so deep down, she did love him. I knew it wasn't the happily-ever-after kind of love, but what she felt for Kal was probably close to the kind of love people bestow upon domestic animals, or their first car.

Dakota wanted to hang onto Kal, even if he wasn't housebroken. So, if I borrowed him for say, three-and-a-half hours of naked bliss, she wasn't likely to forgive me.

Another unsettling thing about my Kal dream was that I thought I hated blond men. Not just Kevin Costner, Willem Dafoe, and Robert Redford, but senators, teachers, and just about any fair-haired man. To have this unbelievably erotic dream about Kal's hands and mouth all over my naked body, and I do mean all over, was just too much. I didn't dare tell a soul that, hidden in my subconscious mind, is an overwhelming desire to play the X-rated version of Twister with Dakota's squeeze. The Freudian implications were astounding.

Despite my sexually deprived state, I was feeling rather pleased about things in a light-hearted, good-humored way. This, of course, was due entirely to Jared. What a fabulous name. It sounds sophisticated and humble at the same time. We'd had lunch every week for the last three weeks. I really enjoyed the lunches, but I was starting to wonder if there was ever going to be any S-E-X in this relationship. He'd kissed me once on the lips, just a quick peck. I could have been his niece. It was a totally asexual, close-mouthed, soft-lipped, peck that made my pulse quicken and my underarms prickle. But it was too brief to ignite anything below my waist. I don't mean to sound ungrateful, because Jared really was very handsome in an extravagantly beautiful, soap-opera star kind of way. And if you add to that his charming and sincere personality, you have a recipe for the perfect guy. Which is why I kept wondering when the fuck were we going to do it?

I knew I was nowhere near as patient as I used to be, but I also knew that when people get along as well as we did, and talked to each other as much as we did, at least an hour every day, they usually wanted to deepen their relationship through sexual exploration.

So why didn't Jared want to explore me? I liked him so much there wasn't anything I didn't like about him. Well maybe one or two things, but they were really minor. And yes, I'd demonstrated my affections to him. I touched his arm, laughed at his jokes. I touched his legs. Once I even brushed my breast against his arm! All I received in return was a thigh caress from his fingers. It was actually a very pleasant sensation because he used his fingers to trace interlocking circles on my bare skin, and the circles kept going higher and higher, until they reached the hemline of my skirt. I was convinced his fingers were going to go all the way up to my pantyline, and perhaps beyond. However, at that point, our lunch arrived and Jared seemed to lose all interest in me once his medium-rare steak was set before him. I guess every guy has his own priorities.

I was going to lunch with Jared again, hoping he had a room booked at the Sutton Place Hotel. Failing that, I hoped we could go to a restaurant where I could have a spicy chicken burger and a strawberry milkshake. I was doubtful about the latter since Jared didn't eat at restaurants that employ teenage managers, and offer kid's toys with their meals.

Jared had a penchant for international cuisine. So far, we'd had food from three different cultures. I was waiting for him to call me, so

I could find out where we'd be eating. I'd dressed up a little more than usual, because I was hoping that day would be sex day. I was wearing a baby blue mini-skirt with a matching jacket. The jacket had sleeves to just beyond my elbows. Underneath, I was wearing a white sleeveless blouse that dipped dramatically at the neck, and hung only as far as my mid-section. When I bent over, the blouse rode up so my back was exposed. Ralph saw this when I was trying to retrieve some papers I'd dropped on my way to the photocopier. He ran his finger along my spine. I must confess it gave me an erotic thrill. Yes, I wanted sex that badly.

Even though I wanted that day to be the big sex day, I wasn't wearing any really sultry underwear. I hadn't bothered to buy any.

I wanted to get a few sexy items that would look like I stepped out of the latest Victoria's Secret catalogue. However, if my relationship with Jared was going to continue as it had so far, I'd have more use for a box of toothpicks and dental floss than a G-string and push-up bra.

When I got back to my desk from the photocopier, the light on my cell phone was blinking. I had a message. I tapped the three numbers on my keypad to retrieve my messages. I had one new message from Jared. We were having Greek food for lunch. I listened as his recorded voice carefully ran through the restaurant's address and directions, and my anticipated time of arrival. He was allowing me time to stare at myself in my compact mirror, run an errand, and circle around looking for the best parking spot. Next, Jared irritated me by requesting that I not arrive at the restaurant late.

He figured he'd accounted for all my distractions, so I was to be punctual. Thus far, I hadn't been more than twelve minutes late for any of our dates. The twelve-minute mishap happened on our second date, when I got lost. I'd been heading in the direction of Bombay Palace, when I remembered I was supposed to meet Jared at Bombay Place. In general, I'd been getting much better at arriving on time. Honest.

Before the message ended, Jared said he was having a hard time concentrating at work, because thoughts of me kept floating through his mind. Wow, that was one of the sweetest things anyone has ever said to me.

I replaced the receiver and let out a sigh so heavy, it ruffled some of the papers on my desk. My emotions were in turmoil. Why wasn't he having thoughts of me sleeping naked in a king-sized bed? Instead he was creating more memories of me eating. This time it was going to be images of me with feta cheese breath and grape leaves caught between my front teeth.

When I arrived at the restaurant, Jared was already seated with a Corona for himself and an iced tea for me. I surprised him by ordering the pork souvlaki, instead of the chicken. He had some lamb thing that I refused to taste.

After we'd eaten, Jared told me he was feeling a knot of tension in his neck and asked if I could do anything about it. A month earlier, I would've had to say no. This past week, however, I started and finished *Massage for Lovers* in four days. I practiced my back massage on Conner. I had to tell him it was part of a martial arts program to get him to comply. I tried my foot massage on Mackenzie, but she kept insisting I was hurting her feet, so I gave up. I was going to try the penis massage on Dogbiscuit, while he was sleeping, but I was afraid he might wake up and kick me in the face, thinking I was a wayward intruder looking for the family jewels.

My first thought when Jared asked me to feel the tension in his neck was, *Hurray, this must be an open invitation to the rest of his body*. After I felt his neck and remarked on its tightness, he asked me to rub out the knot. As I was kneading and pressing and poking, I kept thinking he would place his hands on my thighs and begin caressing my legs. I also thought he might flip me around onto his lap and cradle me like a baby, before carrying me upstairs to the presidential suite. Alas, nothing of the sort happened. First of all, we were in a small Greek restaurant that didn't have an upstairs, let alone a presidential suite. Second, the check arrived and he seemed very anxious to leave. He walked me to my car, something he usually didn't do. Whenever we had a lunch date, we arrived separately and left separately. Once at my car, he invited himself in, and told me we were going someplace.

In the back of my mind, I kept thinking *Park Hyatt here I come*. I'd never stayed there, but I had lots of grand notions of what the rooms were like. If Jared didn't object, I was going to call Dakota from the middle of the bed, after I was replete with the splendor of our glorious lovemaking.

Unfortunately, Jared wan't thinking the same thing I was. His directions were taking us south, not west toward the swank mid-town hotels. We ended up at a farm in the middle of the city. I was starting to feel a bit apprehensive, because I was afraid I might see chickens. Even though I eat chickens, I don't like the sight of live hens walking about. There's something about unplucked, unbutchered, unpackaged poultry that grosses me out. It's the way their heads move while the wings remain motionless. I'm okay if their wings are flapping, but if they aren't, forget it.

Jared must have picked up on my current level of discomfort, because he said, "Don't worry, I'm not going to make you park in the barn with all the livestock."

"That's right, you aren't. Isn't there paved parking around here?" I was driving over a gravel road and my car didn't like it.

"Not where we're going, but it isn't much farther." After a few more twists and turns, we found ourselves surrounded by trees and quiet. No chickens.

"How's that?" Jared asked.

"It's lovely," I said, looking around.

There wasn't a soul in sight. I could hardly believe the farm was just below us, through the bushes and to the left or right. I'd lost all sense of direction. I shut off my car engine. Jared removed his jacket and hung it on the little hook above the rear passenger door. Then he rolled the sleeves of his white shirt up to the elbows. I took off my little jacket and threw it on the back seat. We smiled at each other. I put my hands in my lap and waited for what would come next.

"Now, where were we?" he said, moving over the gearbox. He put his right arm on my shoulder.

"We were heading for the Park Hyatt when we took a wrong turn and ended up here," I said.

"Have you ever done it in a car?"

"No," I said crossing my arms over my chest, frowning.

"Would you like to try?" His voice was warm and seductive. I could feel his breath on my neck.

"I don't know," I said, sulking.

"Sharon, I thought you'd much prefer a romp in the outdoors to..."

"The comforts of a hotel? Bzzzzz! Wrong!" I said, trying to sound like a game-show emcee.

"Don't be this way. I've been trying to restrain myself for weeks, and today, when your gold fingers were touching my neck, I thought I was going to explode."

Wow, what a confession, and he said "gold fingers." I do have gold fingers. Dogbiscuit said the only thing skillful about my hands was the way they never tired of signing credit card receipts. Well, hah! He's wrong. My hands have other talents too.

"Are you mad?" Jared asked. I was tempted to say yes, but you can't stay mad at a person who values your hands that highly.

"No, I'm not mad," I said, "but just so you know for next time, I much prefer a clean bed, fluffy towels, and room service."

"Not all the time," he said, putting his lips on my neck.

"Yes, all the time."

The last word came out as a whisper against his lips. Then I was silenced by the best kiss I'd ever experienced in my life. I know that's not saying a lot, since Jared was only the third man I'd ever kissed, but believe me, it was sensational. I could feel a tingling at the top of my head, and I was sure my panties were drenched. All that, from just one kiss. Jared moved his lips away from mine and smiled at me. He was so handsome, he made my heart do a double-time beat so frantic, it sounded like a personal challenge to the chorus performers from *Lord of the Dance*.

"Has anyone ever touched you like this in a car?" Jared put his hand on my inner thigh and started rubbing.

"No," I said.

"How about like this?" he said, moving his hand up under my skirt. His fingers were making little circles right at the juncture between my legs.

"No," I said. My voice caught in my throat, because his fingers had pushed under my panties. There were no barriers between him and me.

"Has anyone ever done this?" Jared asked, covering my mouth with his so it was impossible for me to answer. Jared lifted his lips from mine again.

"How about this?"

I wanted to say "no". My first attempt came out as a moan. The second time I tried, I ended up saying yes as my hips moved to the rhythm and pace set by Jared's fingers.

"What about this?" His voice was hoarse against my ear. His lips were moving along my neck and over my shoulder.

"What about this," he said, slipping his hands beneath my blouse.

All I was able to say was, "Yes, yes, yes!"

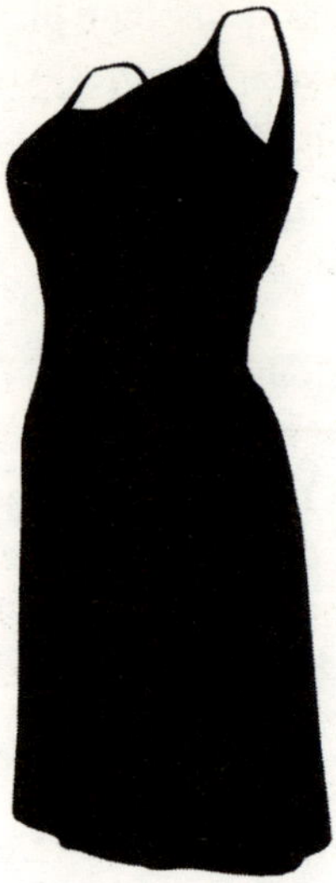

Chapter Ten: *The End?*

Let me just say for the record, I am not the only one with gold fingers. That Greek lunch was the absolute best lunch I ever had. Ever. I know I keep saying that, but oh my God, who could have imagined that in a car, you could enjoy such erotic splendors. I can't believe I've been missing out on these joys all my adult life. Is this the reason teenagers are always so hot to get their hands on the family sedan?

I drove Jared back to the restaurant so he could retrieve his car. He had to direct me again, because I was still very confused and disoriented. Even more so. Rather than telling me in words when to make a left right turn, Jared would caress certain parts of my body, or trace the route on my skin saying, "Go this way" or "Turn here." It made me so excited that twice I almost ran my car up on the curb. Each time, Jared admonished me with a reprimand to focus or concentrate. As if that was going to be possible while he continued his finger play. We made it back to the automated parking lot where Jared had left his car. I drove in and parked right in front of his car's rear bumper.

"Okay, thanks for a great lunch," I said grinning madly. Jared laughed.

"Was it good?" he asked. I wasn't sure if he was asking about the lunch, or the ride up Sugar Mountain. Well, the answer to both questions was the same.

"It was very, very good," I told him, smiling. I didn't think I'd ever stop smiling.

"I'm glad," he said, kissing me on the temple. He took my hands in his, and we sat quietly together for a moment. Then he reached across the seat and kissed me with the same kind of passion you see on soap operas. The only difference was that I think his feelings for me were real and not method acting. When Jared finally lifted his lips from mine, we were both breathing heavily.

"I guess I should go," he said.

I nodded. I couldn't trust my voice.

"Do you want to go to the zoo next week?" he asked, playfully.

"Listen, you," I said, in an admonishing tone I usually saved for Conner and Mackenzie.

"Okay, okay, Park Hyatt it is."

I should have driven myself straight to work, but, I didn't want anything to dampen my happy mood, so I crossed work and home off my destination list. That left malls and boutiques as possible places to spend the rest of the afternoon. I wanted a witness to my happiness, so at the first red light, I pulled out my mobile phone and set up the hands-free earphone. I called Kate. She answered on the first ring.

"Kate McKinley, how may I help you?"

"Hi Kate," I said.

"Hey hon, how are ya?"

"Ex-cell-ent," I said, using my Monty Burns voice.

"You know if you're anything better than fine, I'm going to need to hear all about it."

"I was hoping you would say that," I said. I couldn't wait to tell Kate that I had finally found what I had been looking for all my life. Well, maybe not all my life, but certainly the part of my life that began when I logged onto Ashley Madison. Since that crazy moment of drunken spontaneity, and liquor-supported courage, I'd been looking for something. I felt certain, in the way a good orgasm makes you feel confident, that at last I'd found my missing piece. And now that I had him, I wanted the world to know about my good fortune. Well, not the entire world, because Dogbiscuit and his mom would just freak out if they learned what I'd been up to.

I'd have to keep reminding myself not to rush into the house yelling, "Guess what honey?" Even though I was certain Dogbiscuit wasn't the least bit interested in me sexually, or otherwise for that matter, he wouldn't take kindly to the notion of me finding a super sex cat replacement for him. In my head I kept hearing that song, *No more lonely nights,* something, something, something, something, *wasn't he there for you, didn't he care for you,* something, something, something, something, *No more lonely nights!*

"I'm all ears. Tell me what is been going on," Kate said, breaking into all the thoughts that were screaming in my head.

"I can't have this conversation on a cell," I told her, "Plus I'm driving. Are you busy? Because I was thinking maybe you could meet me for coffee." There was a long pause, the kind that should have been filled with an "um", or an "uh", or a "let me see." Kate's speech is always devoid of such fillers, so all I heard was silence, punctuated by the occasional crackle of telephone static. I could tell Kate's brain was working on her escape plan.

Kate is a managing director for a large headhunter firm that find jobs for the educational elite. Kate's main responsibility is to maintain the huge bank of clients in need of people with specialized skills. This required Kate to do a lot of schmoozing. The result was that she'd become a veritable walking Rolodex of the who's who in town. She knew who did what, for whom, when, and for how long. When it came to networking and building careers, Kate was indispensable. No matter what it was you thought you might want to do, Kate could hook you up with someone who needed you as much as you needed them.

"Where are you?" Kate's voice cut into my thoughts.

"I'm on Bloor," I said.

Prada or Armani?"

"Closer to Armani," I said.

"Let's meet at Hazelton Lanes," she suggested.

"Okay," I said, sailing past Armani, then Chanel. Traffic suddenly stopped moving and I had to crawl past Yves St. Laurent. I had plenty of opportunity to gawk but the windows are always the same, a pile of brown luggage. Can't they get a little more creative?

"How soon will you be there?"

"Soon," I said, turning on my right turn signal.

"Give me fifteen, or twenty minutes," Kate said, jangling something near her phone. Then she hung up. She was probably putting her shoes on and making a grab for her purse at the same time. Like me, Kate often kicked her shoes off when she was at work. I, however, have only ever removed boots, shoes, or a cardigan. Kate, who doesn't have anywhere near the number of issues and inhibitions I do, is likely to kick, push, or slip off any article that restricts or limits her movements. Considering the type of movements Kate enjoys, lots of things might be removed during the course of a day.

Last spring, I stopped by Kate's Bloor Street office because we were going to a networking party at a local bistro. When I arrived on the sixteenth floor, things were pretty quiet. The nine-to-fivers had gone for the day, leaving behind a handful of workhorses, and people from a distant planet who didn't feel compelled to return home each evening, to friends, families, and cable TV. Personally, I think there's something wrong with anyone who stays at work longer than they need to. If my foot doesn't hit the pavement one minute after quitting time, someone better check the elevators because it's highly likely that I'm trapped in one.

When I stepped from the elevator onto that desolate floor, there was no one to herald my arrival. I had to find my way through the maze of cubicles towards Kate's gleaming, but windowless, office. The front of Kate's office is glass. The frosted kind, so that whoever is on the other side remains a deformed mystery until the door opens. I didn't bother peering through the glass. I knocked on the door and waited, and waited. I knocked again, hard, sending a clear message to open the fucking door.

"Come in," called Kate. I opened the door and entered Kate's black leather and chrome office. Kate was sitting on her leather executive chair. She not only had her shoes off, her skirt was unzipped, her blouse was untucked, and her hair was cascading in the wildest waves this side of the Pacific Ocean.

"What are you doing?" I asked.

She looked up at me innocently and said, "I work better this way." When she stood up to hug me, her skirt slipped down to her hips. She caught it and reached around to the back to fasten it.

"Oops," she said, laughing. At first I thought she was tipsy, and I wondered where she was keeping her vodka flask.

"Are you okay?" I asked her, as she straightened herself out, now that her skirt was secure, to her full height of five feet, and ten glorious inches.

"I'm fine. How have you been?" We hugged each other and she smelt of Obsession and felt very soft.

"Where the hell is your bra?" I wailed, loud enough for anyone who overheard to think I'd been the one drinking vodka.

"Right, I had to take that off too. The tension you know? Damn those under-wires."

Kate had a little adjoining closet to her office which she'd always wanted to turn into a powder room, but upper management wouldn't fork out the $20, 000 required by the "Wee, Cheatem and Howe" contracting firm. Personally, I could have gone in there and installed the toilet and pedestal sink in a weekend for a fraction of the quote given by some guy named Joe. I'd seen how to do it on *Designer Renovations*. Anyway, Kate used her little closet as a dressing room/kitchenette. She kept biscotti in the closet along with smart looking Ralph Lauren pumps that hurt her little toes, but looked really rich with her business suits. I thought I heard a ruffling noise in the closet. Kate coughed just as I whipped my head toward the noise. We both looked at the closet.

"What was that?" I asked pointing to the closet.

"My gym bag probably fell over. Just a sec." Kate walked over to the closet and disappeared inside. There were some rummaging sounds, most likely for my benefit. Then there was silence. I waited, not so patiently, by the door. I couldn't look out the front of Kate's office because the frosty glass made it impossible to discern any human shapes. I thought I saw the guy from *Brother From Another Planet* walk by, but I couldn't be sure because the glass made even good-looking people look like alien freaks.

"Okay, ready." Kate gave me her dazzling, cover girl smile. She was totally ready. Her shoes were on and her clothing was set right again. Her hair looked like Moses had calmed it with the same staff he'd used on the Red Sea.

"What were you really doing before I got here?"

"Working," came her chirpy reply. She pushed past me and held her office door open. I walked out and she closed the door firmly.

We went out to the elevators where we had an unusually long wait. We were standing there talking about nothing, when who should happen by? This drop-dead gorgeous twenty-something college intern. He was carrying a jacket, thrown over a fat brief case that made him look like one of those encyclopedia salesmen from the eighties. Although his pants weren't short, they sloshed around his ankles and I noticed he wasn't wearing any socks. He took one look at us, did an about-face, and uttered a quick, "Oops, I forgot something." Yeah, you forgot to wait the fifteen minutes Kate told you to give her so she could clear out without being seen with you. As he made his hasty retreat, I noticed that he had missed two belt loops and his shirt was untucked.

"Who was that?" I asked, using my thumb to point to him in a classic hitchhiker pose. The elevator arrived and Kate launched herself inside. I followed her sedately, and made a point of sticking my head outside the doors of the elevator as if expecting College Boy to join us.

"Get in," Kate ordered. She pressed the Lobby button with her long finger, and kept pressing it, as if it were dispensing ice.

"Who was that guy?" I repeated.

"I don't know," she said, laughing. That made me laugh too.

"What's his name?" I asked. More laughter.

Kate kept shaking her head and laughing.

"Kate, you know him right?"

"He fixes photocopiers." That brought on more hysterical laughter.

"What's his name?" I asked, laughing almost as much as Kate was.

"I don't know. Everyone just calls him Photocopy Guy," she said. That made us both almost fall on the floor, we were laughing so hard. Even though I'm as far from Dr. Ruth as you can get, I know what messy clothes, tussled hair and no socks mean. And no, it doesn't mean the *Miami Vice* look is back.

When we got to the lobby, we were both wiping tears from our eyes. I headed toward the revolving doors and stopped when I realized Kate wasn't with me. I turned around to see her standing as motionless as the Statue of Liberty.

"Kate? What's the matter?" Walking towards her, I saw an odd expression on her face. Something like amused horror.

"I'm not wearing any panties," she said. That sent us both into another fit of hysterical giggles. When I finally recovered, all I could think was, wait till Dakota hears this.

Both Dakota and Kate should have been in *Girls Gone Wild.* One of the few differences between those two is that Dakota tells me everything, almost from the moment it happens. With Kate you have to pry with the same technique you use on a clamshell. When you get her to speak, however, her pearls of information are so wonderfully scandalous, they're worth the effort required to extract them.

Now, my immediate task was getting to Hazelton lanes for my meeting with Kate. I made a right turn onto Avenue Road and drove past the conveniently located and exorbitantly priced Hazelton Lanes parking garage. Anything that costs more than free is expensive parking in my book. I decided to find street parking for the obvious benefit that I wouldn't have to pay five dollars to park my car. When you say it that way, five dollars sounds like a reasonable amount next to a twenty-dollar parking ticket. But I refuse to pay it, on the grounds that I already pay to insure my car. I already pay for a yearly license to drive it. I pay to keep it in good repair, to be washed vacuumed, and air-dried. Add to that the cost of fuel, and five dollars for parking begins to seem a tad excessive. So I find free parking wherever I can, even if I have to burn twenty-two dollars in gas to do it.

Unfortunately, the city's entire populace seemed to have the same idea. I drove around in circles for six minutes. Each time I repeated the loop, my circle became a little wider, and wider still, until I threw in the towel and headed back towards the Hazelton Lanes parking lot. That's when I spotted a smallish spot between an SUV and a minivan. I hate that kind of spot because you have to struggle into it, and getting out is made hazardous because the size of the vehicles surrounding my car creates a blind spot in front and behind me. I was parking in a virtual black hole. Where was my personal driver?

For the moment, all I had to contend with was the getting in. That required all my parking expertise, which isn't a lot. I moved up until I was sitting parallel to the SUV, and then started to back in slowly. I pulled out, pushed back, pulled out, adjusted my angle, pushed back, pushed in some more, then began moving forward made some wheel adjustments and then pushed back again before pulling forward. At last I was in. The whole ordeal reminded me of my first sexual experience with Dogbiscuit. It was painful, annoying, and not something I wanted to repeat. And in both cases, the mirrors were no help.

I practically skipped over to Hazelton Lanes, now that my free parking had been secured. Kate and I had a preferred meeting spot. It was a little kiosk café that had a good selection of teas and an even better selection of pastries. It was more or less in the middle of the mall, so you could enjoy a bite and people-watch with entirely unrestricted views of most of the mall's going and comings.

Kate was nowhere in sight when I arrived. Her office was only a fifteen-minute walk away, but Kate has a far greater propensity for being late than I do. I went to the little kiosk and ordered an Earl Grey tea. I was still pretty full from the pork souvlaki I'd eaten for lunch, but I could handle a butter tart. I decided to hold off on the sweets until Kate arrived, to cutting my calories in half. I was still on my look-great-for-sex diet. Now that it seemed sex was imminent, I had to really hold fast to the fasting. No more cheating. The night before, I'd been really good. I ate an apple just before six. After that, I didn't allow myself anything else. By nine o'clock I was starving. By ten it felt like my stomach had started eating my liver. I went to bed at 10:30, only because I couldn't stand feeling hungry anymore. When I brushed my teeth I piled toothpaste on my brush like it was a buffet selection.

I took my medium-sized tea to a table far enough away from the other two people in the kiosk sitting area. I wanted a table that would allow Kate and I a sense of privacy. Real privacy is too much to hope for in public settings. I know, because I always eavesdrop when I'm out in public. A few times, I've even stopped what I'm doing to listen in on the lives of strangers. I've never interupted, but a few times, I've noticed members of the party involved, directing comments towards me as though I was part of the discussion. Most of the tables had two chairs on opposites sides. I grabbed an extra chair so Kate and I would have a place for our purses. I was just removing the lid from my Styrofoam cup, when she arrived.

"Hi, Sharon," she said, opening her arms for a big hug. I stood up and very carefully stepped into her waiting arms. I didn't want to jostle the table and knock over my tea.

"Oh, you're fully clothed today," I said, with a wink. Kate laughed at my reference to her girl-gone-wild antic of the previous spring.

"So, how are you? Did you ever hear from that guy you were after?"

"First of all Kate, I wasn't after any guy, and second, do you want to split a brownie, butter tart, or slice of banana chocolate fudge cake?"

"Yeah sure. What do you want?"

"I don't know. Everything looks delicious."

From where we were sitting, Kate and I had a completely unrestricted view of the dessert display case.

"Let's order the chocolate brownie cheesecake."

"Okay," I said. I could still remember last night's hunger pangs, so anything sweet was okay with me. Kate went up to the counter to order. In moments, she returned with a coffee, two forks, a napkin, and a generous wedge of cheesecake.

"Wow," I said. "How did you score such a big slice?

"I know the..."

"Never mind," I said. I'm never going to get used to how many people Kate knows. Kate divided the slice perfectly in half. We each took a forkful.

"Mmm," I said.

"Positively orgasmic," Kate said.

"Oh, not quite," I said, smugly.

"Well, aren't you the cat that swallowed the canary."

"Actually, I haven't swallowed anything yet, but I may by next week," I said, coyly.

"Oh my God! Really?"

"Yeah, sure," I said, suddenly feeling shy.

"Tell me everything, name, rank, and serial number." Kate prodded, impatiently pumping her feet under the table. I divulged all of Jared's vital information and waited for her to say "I know him" or "I know his brother's mother-in-law's cousin". But she didn't say anything at all. In fact her face was rapt with attention, so I told her more.

"I met him the same way I met the other guy."

"The one you wanted to call, but thought waiting for him to call was better?"

"Right," I said, although I wasn't sure I ever actually thought that.

"How did you meet?" I was going to say at the Prince Hotel, like you might say I ran into him at the Gap. It wouldn't be lying really, because that is where Jared and I first met face to face. Prior to that he was a faceless, voiceless text message in my Ashley Madison mailbox.

"On the Internet." I finally said, waiting for Kate's eyebrows to rise. They didn't, and there were no signs of her being surprised or alarmed.

"On a dating website, or in a chatroom?"

"Believe it or not, a website for married people," I said.

"I met a guy once at a pub. I knew him from a chat room," Kate replied, oblivious to the gravity of what I'd just told her.

"Really," I said, painfully aware that the conversation was now going to veer sharply away from me and I still had so much more to tell.

"Yes, he was such a sweetheart." Kate had a faraway look in her eyes.

"Did anything happen between the two of you?" I put the last piece of brownie cheesecake in my mouth. It's amazing how quickly half a slice is consumed. Kate was still eating hers.

"We had a brief affair," she said, taking the lid off her coffee.

"How brief?" I asked, knowing how quickly Kate could dispense with men.

"A night and a day," she said, then her face was lost behind the huge Styrofoam cup. She must've ordered a large, and then super-sized it to jumbo.

"Does that qualify as an affair? I've spent more time in the Emergency Room waiting for a doctor to attend to one of my kids' skinned knees."

"Well it's longer than a one-night stand," Kate said adamantly.

"True," I said, nodding, although to me, it seemed like a one-night stand with a complimentary breakfast. Kate finished her cheesecake, then pushed her plate aside.

"Okay," she said, wiping her fingers on a napkin, "your turn. Tell me more about Jared. Is he married?"

"Yes, very married." Was she listening to me at all? "You should see the size of his wedding band."

"Oh, I hate those types," Kate said.

"Cut him some slack, it was probably the wife's idea."

"Sure, but he went along with it."

"Okay, so he doesn't have good taste in wedding bands, and he gives in to his wife's desires. Is that a crime?" I must be in love. I'm defending the man's marriage.

"Well, how bad is her fashion sense?"

"She doesn't have any."

Kate used her hands to muffle her voice and then said, "Houston, we have a problem."

"No, we don't have a problem. He looks great. Nice clothes, perfect teeth, good manners, and—"

"Money?"

"I don't know. Maybe. The important thing is, I like him."

"And he likes you?"

"Yes," I smiled. Kate smiled back.

"Okay, so what have you two done together?" The way Kate said "done," told me she was talking about sex, like, "have you done each other?"

"Just car stuff," I said, taking a drink of tea.

"But not all the way?"

"No, no, no, Kate, I'm not like you." Kate laughed at that and I giggled with her.

"Okay, so now what?"

"Now, I have to get some lingerie, because next week we're having lunch at the Hyatt."

"Nice place, but you don't need lingerie; it's just going to end up in a heap on the floor."

"I am absolutely counting on that, but I want it to be an attractive heap."

"Gotcha," she said taking a sip of coffee.

"Anyway, I think it's a good idea to start each new love relationship with new underwear."

"That's because you married Dogbiscuit. After a while you'll see it's not the packaging, it's the present."

"If that was true, we wouldn't need gift wrapping."

"Good point! You win, we'll go shopping."

The last time I went shopping for lingerie I did a very poor job. I went to all the usual places, Tres Jollie, Melmira, La Vie En Rose, and La Senza. In the last two stores, I decided to buy what the flawlessly beautiful, and impossibly perfect, models were sporting. I know all about airbrushing and computer enhanced busts and leg lengthening, but I still expected to look sexy and, failing that, I thought I'd look nice in my new undies. Sadly, I didn't. Dogbiscuit confirmed this when he spotted them.

"What the devil are you wearing?" he asked.

"These are new and they were very expensive, so I won't take kindly to anything negative said about them."

"I wasn't going to say anything about them, it's you that has the problem."

"What problem might that be?" I don't know why I didn't just keep my mouth shut.

"Well, on you, those wretched things look like hospital bandages."

"Hospital bandages?" I'd never felt so insulted.

"Yes," he said, sneering wickedly at me.

"Well, I guess I should just take them off then."

"That might not be a bad idea. Anyone who sees you like that, is likely to start rubbing Polysporin all over your ass."

In retrospect, I should've known better. Anyone else would've purchased items that flattered their physique. Rather unfortunately, I somehow managed to buy panties that looked like coverings for a burn victim. Kate assured me that my past mistakes were not going to be repeated.

"Yes, but I don't want to make any new mistakes either," I told her. She assured me that she had a foolproof method to assist me in dressing for sexual conquest. Kate said my first mistake was going north of Bloor Street.

On Saturday, we headed south. Kate took me to that part of town acclaimed for trendy eateries. The same neighborhood is frequented by pushers, pimps, and prostitutes. To say there's never a dull moment in that part of town, would be overstating the obvious. The shop Kate led me to was the Wal-Mart of the sex trade. Everything you can imagine was there, in addition to stuff that defied belief.

The sex shop was mind bending, thrilling, and full of surprises at every turn. It was like something from an amusement park. Of course, I'd expected the crude assortment of crotchless panties, and anatomically correct dildos, but the shop had so much more. I could hardly keep myself from gushing, "Kate look at this!" There were a million gadgets, gizmos, and accessories. By accessories I don't mean necklaces and handcuffs. This store went far beyond that. I found some adhesive stars that were perfect for my nipples. Kate actually purchased a leather and chain contraption that did something to a woman's clitoris. It looked so painful, I was afraid to ask what it did. If I ever tried to put something like that on, I'd probably need to be rescued. I couldn't imagine the humiliation of dialing 9-1-1 with my big toe, not to mention the look on the faces of the paramedics when they arrived to rescue me.

Kate and I spent almost two hours in the sex shop. When we finally filed through the cash desk, I forked over $260 in exchange for a few flimsy items, none of which was big enough to cover a sneeze. Do men have to put this kind of effort into preparing for sex? When I asked Kate, she gave me the look and then asked if I wanted to try a Brazilian wax. I liked Jared a lot, but I wasn't sure I liked him enough to endure that kind of pain.

That Friday, I started getting ready for my date with Jared as soon as Dogbiscuit left for work. I was nervous and excited and worried that he wouldn't like my underwear. I thought it was exceptionally pretty. It was white and really delicate. It looked like it was made from sewing together the petals of small flowers. There was lots of exposed skin to excite Jared's senses. Hopefully.

Jared asked me to meet him early so we could have a few hours together. I was supposed to meet him at 11 and I actually arrived at the Park Hyatt at 11:03. A personal best.

"How did you do it?" Jared asked me when we were secured in room 1212.

"I realized that the later I am, the less time I'll have with you," I told him truthfully.

In return for my honesty, I received the best kiss ever. Jared just keeps getting better and better. The more time I spend with him, the more time I want to spend with him. Is this what they call love? I'd spent most of the week fantasizing about what it was going to be like to be naked with Jared. Of course, I thought he'd look amazing and everything would be splendid, and I would have the biggest, and best orgasm ever. And when things turned out better than I'd imagined,

I almost fainted with joy.

Afterward, Jared held me close to his chest, our hands and legs entwined. My eyes were closed and I was about to drift off to sleep, when I heard his voice faintly in my ear. Jared's voice was just above a whisper, but what he said was so shocking, it was as if he'd shouted. "I love you, Sharon."

And in that instant, my heart grew three sizes, just like the Grinch's. When I closed my eyes a second time, I could no longer see the beautiful room, but I continued to feel the heat from Jared's strong arms, and I could hear the deep thump of his heart. I felt all the stress drain from my body. My long and arduous odyssey was over, and I could relax. I'd always been a worrier. I worried about my looks, my social life, my marriage, my job, what people thought of me, what they were saying, the future, the present, money. You name it. But cradled in his embrace, I felt as if just having Jared next to me was all I'd ever need. I experienced a feeling so profound and so great, I can only call it Bliss.

Bonjour! Je suis tres heureuse. I've been trying to speak only in French since Dakota and I arrived in Paris last week. Even though I lost the bet we'd made before I met Jared, Dakota thought I deserved the trip. I agreed. We only came for the weekend, but we're still here. *Je ne veux pas depart.* I don't want to go back home. Neither does Dee. If it weren't for Mackenzie and Connor, I might stay. I could start a new life here.

Dakota has been looking at flats. We looked at three on Tuesday. I thought we were apartment hunting to keep out of the shops, but now it seems that Dakota was serious. I don't think she's going to return with me. She says she has nothing to go back to. Kal calls her everyday, but it doesn't help. For one thing, he's making long-distance calls on Dakota's phone. He told her he was going to start a business, a real business as a handyman. I thought that was a great idea. Dakota says he isn't handy. At least not in the traditional sense of the word handyman. Anyway, I think Kal is serious. I think he really loves Dakota and he's willing to get off his ass to prove it. Dakota just says, "We'll see."

I'm reluctant to go home because I have to face some huge decisions. For one thing, Dogbiscuit and I can't continue as we have been. I don't love him and he doesn't love me. That alone is enough to make me consider ending the marriage. Add to that the fact that I actually want to be in a healthy loving relationship and there seems to be only one course of action. I've always been afraid of divorce because I thought it would be harmful to my kids. However, I now think living this kind of lie is more harmful. I don't want Mackenzie to have a husband like Dogbiscuit. I don't want Connor to treat his wife or girlfriend the way Dogbiscuit treats me. When I was getting ready for this trip, I realized that my children have never once seen me bestow a single act of affection on Dogbiscuit. Never a kiss, nor a romantic embrace. Not even a hug. For his part, Dogbiscuit never speaks to me. To him, I'm an intrusion on his life, and a financial liability that needs to be minimized. When I consider all this, I wonder what impression will be left on my children. I cringe at the thought that years from now Mackenzie and Connor might study the relationship between Dogbiscuit and I as an example of what not to do in a marriage. Wrong or right, I actually believe I have an obligation to show my children what a healthy adult relationship looks like. It doesn't look like what Dogbiscuit and I have now. And without love or commitment to each other, there's no hope for a future together.

That's why I've decided to file for divorce when I return. It makes me sad, because although Dogbiscuit hasn't been much of a dad, he has been around. He hasn't always been dead weight as Dakota claims. My kids are going to have a hard time getting used to his absence. And then again, maybe they won't. There's always the telephone for weeknight chats, and the weekends for outings. Divorce doesn't have to be all bad. Maybe once he's separated from them, he'll feel a greater need to be active in their lives. It could happen.

As for me, I'm ready to start a better life. Of course I want Jared to be part of that life, but he is so married. Before I left for Paris, he told me again that he loves me. I know he means it. He even says he's going to leave his wife. Kate says not to hold my breath. While Dakota and I were boarding the plane for our Parisian mini-holiday, I told her that Jared had said he loved me. She didn't say anything. She just rolled her eyes, and ushered me into J-class. The stewardess handed me a glass of champagne and before long I was far too giddy to bother fighting with Dakota about Jared. I know she wants me to be cautious to avoid getting hurt, but I'm a good judge of character. Never mind the mistake I made marrying Dogbiscuit. I was young and foolish then. Maybe I am still.

However, now I don't feel so empty. I no longer feel like I need to have certain conditions met before I can allow myself to love someone. Now I feel like I can love unconditionally. It was Jared who helped me attain this level of enlightenment. I want to spend the rest of my life learning from him, because in so many ways I feel my journey in this life has just begun.

I know a life with Jared wouldn't be free from pain, and frustrations, or trials and traumas. He isn't a saint, but I love him anyway. And that's essentially the problem I had in my relationship with Dogbiscuit. I couldn't love him, even when I tried.

I wish Jared had come to me under different circumstances. Maybe when were both divorced and vacationing in Freeport, or Montego Bay. But he came to me via the Internet with a wife and a child and a strong desire to do the right thing.

I know it seems impossible for two married people to meet, fall in love, divorce their respective spouses, and then marry each other, but it could happen. The question is, could it happen to me? Can Jared and I be a modern-day Mike and Carol Brady? I don't want to seem juvenile about such serious life-altering circumstances, but I think I love Jared. We've only been together for about eight months, but when he holds my hand, and I look into his eyes, I'm overcome by the strength of my feelings for him. I can't help believing that in all of this there lies waiting for me a happily-ever-after ending. I don't know how long it will take me to get there, but at least I know where I'm headed.

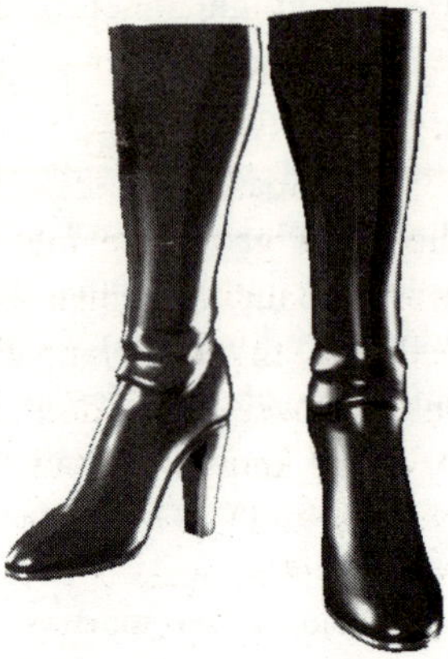

Epilogue

It's been fourteen months since I made my last diary entry. It was certainly a very event-filled time. Jared and I are no longer seeing each other romantically. He and his wife were able to sort things out and fix their relationship, so we decided to cool it, but we still keep in touch and remain very good friends. Jared credits the sense of relaxed, well-being he got from our time together, as well as the discussions we had about our respective difficulties with helping him put his own marriage in perspective. I miss the closeness we shared, but I understand. It was a little sad, but I wouldn't have missed my time with Jared for anything. It might have been brief and it might have been extremely unconventional by public standards, but it was love just the same, and Jared and I were both very happy. Anyway, I haven't had time to mope about it. I've had so many other wonderful experiences with other guys on the site. Some I met, others I chatted with.

As for my own marriage, I'm now separated from Dogbiscuit. I've accepted that we're simply not meant to be and should never have rushed into marriage, especially under the circumstances in which we did.

The split has been amicable and in some ways, our relationship is better now. Since he moved out, he's been much more attentive to the kids. Where he was once distant and detached, he's become really committed to spending his allotted time with them as best he can. Quality time, he calls it, and he truly means it. We've both developed an appreciation for each other's needs and a sincere respect for what the other is going through.

Ironically, now that we're apart, I'm seeing Dogbiscuit in a whole new light. After all the other guys I've met on Ashley Madison, I've come to realize my understanding of men was so limited when we hooked up all those years ago, that our compatibility problems were just as much my fault as they were his. I don't know if we'd still be together if I knew then what I know now, but I'm confident I would have done things differently with Dogbiscuit and it probably would've been less strained. As it is, I'm glad my feelings for him have mellowed and become more affectionate. Hell, I don't even call him Dogbiscuit anymore. I actually refer to him by his given name when talking about him to my girlfriends. It's Kenneth.

I've learned a lot more about life and people in the last year, but more than that, I've learned a lot more about myself. I've come to terms with my own flaws. Flaws I might never have become aware of, had I continued to live such a sheltered existence. I'm no longer on the Ashley Madison site because, since I'm no longer attached, I figure it wouldn't be right if I continued to portray myself that way. You can call what I've done an adventure, an odyssey, or a journey of discovery. It doesn't matter what you call it. What matters is that I went on it.

I hope this recounting of my experiences is considered entertaining in some way. I'd be very happy if it proved helpful to anybody in similar circumstances. When I was writing it, I was just looking for an outlet for my thoughts and emotions to a surrogate confessor. Now that my Ashley Madison adventures are over and I've been convinced to publish these memoirs (convinced by, guess who, Dakota, of course) I must admit, I'm a little jazzed at the notion of so many people reading what was once a confidential diary. It's a bit of a cathartic thrill.

I don't know what the future will hold for me, but I do know that I'm better equipped to handle whatever comes my way and, good or bad,

I'm confident I'll grow from it. While it's true an unexamined life is not worth living, I've discovered it's more important to remember that an unlived life is not worth examining.

Sharon "Sharalike"